YOUR 30 DAY
heart smart
SOLUTION

by Lorna R. Vanderhaeghe

First published in Canada in 2009 by
Headlines Promotions Ltd.

Reprinted and revised in January 2014 by
Lorna Vanderhaeghe Health Solutions, Inc.

Copyright © Lorna R. Vanderhaeghe

All rights reserved. The use of any part of this publication
reproduced, transmitted in any form or by any means,
electronic, mechanical, recording or otherwise, or stored in
a retrieval system, without the prior consent of Headlines
Promotions Ltd. is an infringement of copyright laws.

ISBN: 978-0-9731803-6-7

Cover by BbM Graphics
Interior book design by BbM Graphics
Edited by Krista Belli

DISCLAIMER: While all care is taken with the accuracy of
the facts and procedures in this book, the authors accept
neither liability nor responsibility to any person with
respect to loss, injury or damage cause, or alleged to be
caused directly or indirectly, by the information contained
in this book. The purpose of this book is to educate and
inform. For medical advice, you should seek the individual,
personal advice and services of a health-care professional.

Those wishing to obtain additional copies of this book
or requesting permission to reproduce material from it
may contact:
Lorna Vanderhaeghe Health Solutions, Inc.
106A – 3430 Brighton Avenue
Burnaby, BC V5A 3H4
E-mail: admin@hormonehelp.com

Printed and bound in Canada

Contents

Introduction 1

All About the Heart 5

Heart Disease Risks 15

The Lowdown on Cholesterol and Blood Pressure 24
    Cholesterol 24
    Triglycerides 28
    Lipoprotein(a) and Apolipoprotein B 28
    Homocysteine: Too Much of a Good Thing 29
    High Iron is Dangerous 30
    Fibrinogen: Blood Clot Indicator 31
    C-reactive Protein: Inflammation Agent 32
    High Blood Pressure 34

Diabetes and Depression: Double Trouble 37
    Not Sweet for the Heart 38
    Lifestyle Is the Best Drug 39
    Diabetes Prevention 40
    Heart Disease Linked to Depression 41
    Women More at Risk 42
    Anger Hurts the Heart 45

Heart-Smart Personal Assessment 47

The Heart-Smart Diet 51
    What Is a Carbohydrate? 51
    Hearts Love Fiber 52
    Fat Phobia 56
    Unsaturated Fats: Not Just Good but Fabulous 60
    Omega-3 Superstars 62
    Docosahexaenoic acid (DHA) 64
    Sound Cardiology Advice 67
    The Protein Difference 68
    Eat Like a Mediterranean 70
    Powerful Pomegranate 72
    Dangerously Sugary Drinks 73

The Sodium-Potassium Connection 75
Multipurpose Heart Mineral 76

Heart-Smart Nutrients 79
Sytrinol Lowers Cholesterol in 30 Days & Keeps Arteries Clear 80
Sytrinol Is a Powerful Antioxidant & Improves Cholesterol 81
Sytrinol's Top Five Actions Maintain a Healthy Heart 82
Pine Bark Extract Protects the Heart 86
Pine Bark Extract Lowers High Blood Pressure 87
Pine Bark Extract – Blood Clot Preventer 87
Pine Bark Extract Repairs Capillaries 88
Pine Bark Extract Prevents Fat Deposition in Artery Walls 89
Coenzyme Q10 – The Heart Superstar 89
Statin Drugs Deplete CoQ10 & Increase Breast Cancer Risk 90
CoQ10 Lowers Blood Pressure 91
Cardiovascular Benefits of CoQ10 92
Marvelous Magnesium 93
Potassium and Sodium Need Magnesium 94
Magnesium Protects Against Stroke 94
Magnesium Lowers Bad Cholesterol While
   Increasing Good Cholesterol 94
Magnesium Regulates Blood Pressure 95
Multivitamins and Minerals to the Rescue 96
Hard Arteries and Vitamin K2 98

How to Tame Stress 101
Why We Need to De-stress 104
Deep Breathing for Relaxation 104
Yoga: Ancient Practice Has Heart 105
Meditate Stress Away 105
Stress and the Adrenal Connection 106
Herbs to Reduce Stress 107
Do You Live with Heart? 109
Laughter: The Best Medicine 110
Self-honesty: Emotions and Expression 111
Other Important Heart-Smart Tips 111

References and Resources 114

chapter one

Introduction

Nobody suspected that Grandma Ruby had heart problems until she collapsed on Christmas Day while preparing dinner. To her family and friends, she'd always seemed invincible. A tireless housekeeper never without a dishcloth in her hands or a leaf blower hoisted on her back. A seasoned cook who spoiled guests with enough food to feed half the neighborhood. Even Ruby might not have suspected that she had heart disease, a condition that affects millions of North Americans. With a hardworking mentality, she probably would have treated symptoms like breathlessness and tightness in the chest as an annoyance, as something to bear, not worth seeing a doctor for. Tragically, had she sought help earlier and taken more proactive measures, she might have lived past her mid-70s.

There is a Grandma Ruby in everybody's life – a best friend, a coworker, a partner, a cousin, or a sibling who is diagnosed with heart disease. Heart disease afflicts one in three Americans. In Canada, a heart attack or stroke kills someone every seven minutes. The bulk of heart disease deaths are in women. Women are more likely to die of a heart attack than of breast cancer – a surprising fact to many. For decades, the mental image of a red-faced man clutching his chest has dominated the media. However, we're now realizing – and publicizing – that due to a variety of factors, women are just as vulnerable as men to diseases of the cardiovascular system.

Cardiovascular disease is an umbrella term for diseases and injuries of the heart (including valve and rhythm issues), heart failure, diseases of the blood vessels and stroke.

Startling Statistics
- Every 37 seconds, an American dies of cardiovascular disease (CVD).
- About 80,000,000 American adults (one in three) have one or more types of CVD.
- Every seven minutes, someone in Canada dies from heart disease or stroke.
- CVD accounts for one-third of Canadian deaths.
- About 70,000 heart attacks occur each year in Canada, resulting in 19,000 deaths.

Until the age of 40, women have lower rates of cardiovascular disease than men (eight versus 16 percent). From ages 40 to 80, the rate of cardiovascular disease in both sexes levels off, at about 73 percent. But by the time they reach 80, the rates for women surpasses that of men by seven percent (86 versus 79 percent). The lifetime risk for cardiovascular disease is two in three for men, and more than one in two for women at age 40.

Did You Know...

Every year since 1900, except for 1918, cardiovascular disease (including heart disease) has claimed the same number of lives as cancer, chronic lower respiratory diseases, accidents and diabetes mellitus combined, according to the American Heart Association.

Prevention Intervention
Although heart disease is a leading killer, there is an upside. Heart disease is preventable – and reversible. Like other progressive diseases such as diabetes and cancer, it doesn't have to result in

millions of patients who clutter hospitals, fill drug prescriptions and require expensive operations. No matter what our age, regardless of whether we're 19 or 90, we can strengthen our hearts. We have the power within ourselves to make educated choices about diet, lifestyle, exercise and supplements, and our bodies will reward us with disease-free vitality.

Diet is the first pillar of heart health. However, maybe "diet" is the wrong word. Diet implies changing our eating habits for a designated period of time. Eating for your heart means making long-term changes with regards to what's on your plate and in your glass. You don't want to be like most people who change their diet only upon diagnosis of a disease. Be proactive. By eating the Heart-Smart way, you'll also provide the body with nutrients and protective elements it needs to prevent and alleviate other degenerative ailments.

Related to diet is nutritional supplementation. Is supplementing really necessary, you might ask, if you're already doing everything else? The answer is a resounding yes. Specific nutrients have been shown to have a markedly beneficial effect on ailing hearts, high cholesterol and blood pressure. Even late-stage heart disease and post-surgery conditions can benefit from vitamins, minerals and nutrients such as magnesium, coenzyme Q10, sytrinol, pine bark extract and essential fatty acids.

Physical activity is another big component of any heart health program. A sedentary lifestyle weakens the heart and disrupts blood sugar levels, immunity, mental health and hormones. Conversely, getting fit is the cheapest and most effective therapy for overall health improvement. Although we don't dwell on exercise in this booklet, read about a quick and daily Heart-Smart exercise program in *Heart Smart for Women and the Men They Love.*

No heart book is complete without a discussion of stress reduction and management. Many risk factors for heart disease are exacerbated by stress. Stress itself is toxic for the heart; related to stress is anxiety. Often panic attacks are mistaken for heart attacks, highlighting this very fundamental connection. There are various anti-stress and mental/emotional health strategies that play a valuable role in heart disease prevention and treatment.

Your heart will thank you for picking up this book because it means you're interested in making life changes. Maybe you've recently received a diagnosis you didn't like. Maybe your cholesterol readings having been climbing for years but now they're dangerously high. Maybe you have a strong family history of heart disease that you want to head off at the pass. It's never too early, or too late, to think about how to strengthen your hard-working heart. By combining a heart-healthy diet and key nutritional supplements with exercise and stress reduction strategies, you'll quickly begin to feel better and more vibrant.

chapter two

All About the Heart

Cardiovascular problems can affect not only heart function but also that of the blood vessels running throughout the body. This is why we often see cardiovascular issues in the brain, lungs and lower extremities too. By far, the most common type of cardiovascular disease is coronary artery disease. It's technically a disease of the arteries, the passageways that deliver blood to the needy heart muscle. If blood flow is restricted or blocked, the result is ischemic heart disease. *Ischemic* means "insufficient blood and oxygen flow to the body's tissues" in Latin. Common symptoms include chest pain (angina) and/or heart attack.

Our Powerful Pump
Clench your fist and there you have the approximate shape and size of your heart muscle, nestled in behind your breastbone. The heart has four chambers – two upper (atria) and two lower (ventricles). Oxygen-depleted, bluish blood that has passed through the body collects in the right atrium, then flows down into the right ventricle. From there, it's pumped via the pulmonary artery to the lungs, where it picks up fresh oxygen. The now re-oxygenated, bright red blood travels through the pulmonary veins back into the heart, but this time, it flows into the left atrium, and then down into the left ventricle. Finally, it leaves the heart through the aorta to begin its next cycle journeying throughout the body.

What a process! The heart beats an average 100,000 times a day. Day in, day out, from birth to death (upwards of 2.5 billion heartbeats), the blood delivers oxygen, nutrients, hormones and other important constituents to every cell in our body. At the same time, it collects cellular junk – the unwanted waste of regular processes that occur inside cells. Think of this mighty heart muscle as the pump that keeps everything else running. Just like a mechanical pump needs fuel to keep working, the heart requires a steady supply of blood and oxygen to stay healthy. Problems arise when it doesn't get this fuel because of the fact that, somewhere in the system, a blockage has occurred.

Our Artery Helpers
The heart has two major arteries: the right coronary artery and the left main coronary artery. Each of these arteries stretches out into smaller and smaller arteries, delivering blood deeper into the heart muscle cells. If the blockage develops in one of these arteries, we call it atherosclerosis from the Greek *athere* (meaning "porridge") and *sclerosis* (meaning "hardening" or "scarring"). Over time, plaque builds up on the arterial walls and causes them to stiffen. This accumulation narrows the arteries, and blood clots sometimes form on top of the plaque. The result is reduced blood flow through the heart. If blood flow stops completely, a heart attack (or myocardial infarction, meaning "death of heart tissue") occurs.

By far, the most common reason for reduced blood flow to the heart is atherosclerosis. However, there are other possible reasons for blocked arteries. Blood could be too thick, for instance. Ideally, blood is thin so it can pass unheeded through increasingly miniscule passageways on its way to and from cells. Sometimes, red blood cells have to bend and squeeze through single file because the arterial tunnel is so tiny! But when we, say, eat too much fatty food, that fat ends up in the blood and clogs it up. Blood thickens and the cells also clump together if the body's clotting factors are affected. Our poor circulation then slows while the heart is forced to work harder to counteract the effects of fatty blood. Sometimes, the reason behind diminished blood flow lies with the heart muscle itself. Maybe it has been weakened or damaged as a result of a previous heart attack. The left ventricle, which pumps freshly oxygenated blood back into the body, is particularly relevant to heart disease. Uncontrolled high blood pressure can cause poor left ventricle function and worsen heart disease.

Clogged Pipes

Far from being an inanimate pipe, your arteries are very much a player in this inner game of life. They contract and expand in response to pressure. Arteries have three layers: the outer, tougher adventitia, the middle smooth-muscle media and an inner layer (intima) that's lined with a single layer of specialized cells called the endothelium. This last ultra-thin barrier is a key component in the development of atherosclerosis.

Besides their ability to gauge blood pressure and flow, these multi-functioning endothelial cells interact with substances carried by blood, produce compounds that affect cell growth, and help govern muscle tone, thus allowing arteries to expand and contract to push blood along. Unfortunately, the endothelial layer frequently gets injured. The possible causes are many, including physical force and high blood pressure. Blood also carries toxins (environmental, dietary, metabolic), fatty proteins, excess blood sugar (glucose), infectious microbes and unhealthy cholesterol. All of these can cause endothelial dysfunction and trigger the chain of events leading to atherosclerosis, high blood pressure, heart attack, stroke, and heart failure.

The Role of Cholesterol

Cholesterol has gotten a bad wrap. Our body produces cholesterol, a waxy, fatty substance, to perform a number of important functions.

It is the building block of cellular membranes and is needed to make bile acids so we can digest and absorb our food, as well as to make vitamin D and hormones. To move through the bloodstream, cholesterol puts on a protective coat of lipoprotein particles: low-density lipoprotein (LDL), the "bad" cholesterol, and high-density lipoprotein (HDL), the "good" cholesterol. Generally, we want to keep LDL cholesterol levels down to prevent it from lodging in arterial walls. Conversely, we want higher levels of HDL cholesterol, which protect the heart by sweeping LDL cholesterol through the arteries towards the liver, where it's processed, and then excreted from our system.

♡ Dietary Versus Blood Cholesterol

Have you ever been told to avoid eggs because they are a "high cholesterol" food? This advice stems from a misunderstanding about the difference between dietary and blood cholesterol. Dietary cholesterol is in food, whereas blood cholesterol is made by the body and found in the bloodstream. Eating foods containing dietary cholesterol, however, won't necessarily put cholesterol into the bloodstream. Blood cholesterol is made in the liver from fats, sugars and proteins. The more processed foods, refined oils and sugars you consume, the more cholesterol is produced. Free radical damage also causes the body to produce more cholesterol because cholesterol is used to repair damaged cells, tissues and organs.

Studies show that eggs won't increase cholesterol levels and may actually help lower them. Eggs contain lecithin, which emulsifies the cholesterol in them. Homogenized milk does more damage to arteries than eggs ever will because the fat globules in it have been mechanically altered to such a small state that they can be absorbed directly into the bloodstream.

A low-glycemic, unprocessed, healthy-fat diet is key to cholesterol reduction, and fiber is absolutely critical as it locks onto excess cholesterol and helps eliminate it. For recommendations, see page 51.

When endothelial cells are damaged, they trigger an immune response. The body sends in a repair team to address the inflamed injury, but other scroungers also show up: blood fats and bad LDL cholesterol. Now, rather than help with repairs, immune cells begin an overzealous inflammatory process. As they migrate into the artery wall to help the injury, they ingest the LDL cholesterol and form bloated, fatty foam cells that end up becoming atherosclerosis plaque. The damage is worse if the LDL cholesterol is oxidized, i.e. previously damaged by free radicals. Oxidized LDL cholesterol also damages neighboring cells at the injury site in a chain-reaction-type effect.

Free Radicals and Antioxidants

Think of rust for a minute. Slowly but surely, various chemical reactions occur and the result is an invasive corrosion that is the bane of every vehicle owner's existence! The damage created by free radicals in the body is like rust. Free radicals are a natural byproduct of everyday reactions that produce energy for the body. Other major sources and generators include:
• Fried foods and heated oils
• Nitrates and nitrites in meats
• Toxic airborne chemicals
• Cigarette smoke, or smoke from forest fires
• Exposure to medical or electromagnetic radiation
  (ie. computer terminals)
• Strenuous exercise
• Chlorinated water
• A high-fat diet
• Prolonged physical and/or emotional stress.

What these tiny molecules lack in size, they make up in destructive capacity. Many free radicals are highly toxic, mutagenic (cause cells to mutate) and carcinogenic (cause cancer). Stable molecules are held together by two electrons, but free radicals are missing one electron that they thus attempt to steal from neighboring molecules. An undesirable ripple effect occurs in which more damage is created to others molecules in cells and cell membranes, and more free radicals are formed. Eventually, if left unattended, what was once comparable to a spot of rust becomes a car riddled with unsightly holes.

The progression of free radical damage can, fortunately, be kept in check with antioxidants from our food and nutritional supplements. Antioxidants are free radical scavengers. They readily disable free radicals, preventing healthy body tissues from being damaged. When the body is deficient in antioxidants, our risk of disease increases and aging accelerates. By eating foods rich in antioxidants such as vitamins A, C, and E, selenium and phytochemicals (the pigments that give plants their colors), we can keep our defenses against free radicals strong and stave off their heart-unfriendly effects. Supplemental pine bark extract, sytrinol and coenzyme Q10 serve the same important function and further protect against heart disease via other mechanisms that we'll discuss later.

When Plaque Ruptures

As atherosclerosis progresses, arterial plaque grows and hardens as more cholesterol is absorbed into the artery wall along with other fats and inflammatory cells. Over this, a kind of cap forms, some big, some small. Smaller plaques are thought to be more dangerous due to their greater tendency to rupture in response to a variety of physical and emotional triggers. When this happens, the immune system erroneously orders the production of factors that dissolve the plaque cap, causing its contents to spill back into the artery. Another immune response kicks in, attracting blood platelets. They clump together around the ruptured plaque and, along with red blood cells and other clotting factors, form a blood clot. If that blood clot fully blocks a coronary artery, a heart attack results.

How tragic that the first symptom of heart disease to be taken seriously is usually a heart attack and, sometimes, death! The problem often lies in our general disconnect from our body. We're under such stressors in daily life that we miss or disregard warning signs like chest pain, which occurs when coronary arteries narrow by about 50 percent. Medically termed *angina* (Latin for "squeezing of the chest"), symptoms include:

- Pain radiating from the chest that spreads to your left arm, neck, back, throat or jaw
- Tightness, pressure, squeezing and/or aching in your chest or arm(s)
- Persistent sensation of moderate to severe indigestion
- Sharp, burning or cramping pain
- An ache starting in, or spreading to, your neck, jaw, throat, shoulder, back or arm(s)
- Neck or upper back discomfort, particularly between the shoulder blades
- Numbness in your arms, shoulders or wrists.

Women with angina are more likely to notice abdomen, shoulder and back discomfort than men. Likewise with actual heart attacks, symptoms vary between the sexes. Women are also more likely than men to suffer silent heart attacks, and to report experiencing symptoms up to a month prior to a heart attack.

♡ Heart Attack Symptoms

FOR MEN AND WOMEN

- Episodes of angina (chest pain) that increase
- Uncomfortable pressure, squeezing, tightness, fullness or burning ache in the chest
- Pain or discomfort that radiates to the shoulders, arms, neck, upper back, or jaw
- Shortness of breath
- Sweating, nausea, fainting and dizziness

FOR WOMEN

- Unusual fatigue that worsens with activity, tiredness or depression
- Chest cramping or dull chest pain, as if you have pulled a muscle from the center of your back to your chest
- Heartburn, lower gastric pain or feeling of indigestion
- Overall feeling of weakness or illness
- Feeling like a rubber band is constricting your throat
- Paleness, profuse sweating
- Sleep disturbances

In the case of a heart attack or symptoms leading up to it, the sooner medical attention is sought, the greater your chances of avoiding heart damage. The longer blood supply is impeded or cut off, the more damage the heart potentially sustains. After 20 to 40 minutes, damage can be irreversible. Living tissue becomes scar tissue. Sadly, women are more likely to brush off warning signs, perhaps fearing embarrassment. When women do get a diagnosis and treatment, it usually occurs when they are older and heart disease is more advanced. Sadly, women are also more likely than men to drop out of cardiac rehabilitation programs after a heart attack.

Other Heart Conditions

■ *Arrhythmias*

Usually, the heart beats 60 to 100 times per minute with the same lapse between each beat. Arrhythmia represents an irregular rhythm. There are several types of arrhythmia with varying in degrees of dangerousness. Some are linked to underlying heart disease and others to low thyroid, iron deficiency, anemia and stress. Ventricular tachycardia and ventricular fibrillation are two potentially fatal kinds. In atrial fibrillation, another type which occurs in one percent of people over the age of 60, the heart seems to quiver instead of beating regularly because electrical impulses have been disturbed. If the underlying causes of arrhythmia are treated, they often settle down on their own.

■ Valve Disorders

With mitral stenosis, the heart's mitral valve has a narrowed opening that restricts blood flow from the left atrium into the left ventricle. Shortness of breath results when blood pressure builds up in the atrium and affects the lungs. If the valve develops a leak, blood flows backwards into the heart chamber, requiring the heart to work harder and, over time, possibly resulting in heart failure. Causes of a leak include mitral valve prolapse, infectious bacteria and a damaged heart muscle.

In aortic stenosis, a narrowed aortic valve reduces blood flow from the heart to the rest of the body. The left ventricle enlarges due to the strain, possibly resulting in angina or faintness. If left unrepaired by surgery, congestive heart failure and death may result. The aortic valve can also develop a leak, eventually causing heart failure if untended.

■ Heart Failure

When the heart muscle is weak, damaged and/or abnormally thick, it becomes an inefficient pump. The result is insufficient blood flow to the body that leads to heart failure. As the body tries to compensate, symptoms include a higher heart rate, increased blood pressure and fluid retention. As the current population living with heart disease rises, so does the incidence of heart failure. Acute heart failure occurs when the heart suddenly stops pumping efficiently. Blood backs up in the pulmonary veins, and the pressure causes the lungs to fill with fluid (pulmonary edema), creating an emergency situation.

The most common cause of heart failure is coronary artery disease, and it usually occurs after one or more heart attacks and resultant high blood pressure. Other causes include valvular heart disease, inflammatory viruses and diseases, and damage caused by alcohol and drug use. Symptoms include swelling (edema) of the legs, feet or abdomen, shortness of breath, a nighttime cough, fatigue, chest pain and pressure, weight gain and dizziness. Keep in mind that not everyone with progressive heart failure exhibits symptoms.

Interestingly, we now know that heart failure differs between the sexes. In men, it is more often due to systolic dysfunction, meaning that the heart is weakened, enlarged and can't sufficiently pump blood throughout the body. This is often referred to as a "floppy heart." Women, meanwhile, have what is described as a "stiff heart" that is associated with diastolic dysfunction, meaning that the heart's ability to relax between beats is impaired. A stiff heart muscle is small and cannot fill normally with blood. Regardless of whether your heart is floppy or stiff, heart failure is treatable and should be monitored.

The expression "Prevention is a pound of cure" applies to no condition better than to heart disease. By taking proactive steps to address the risk factors we can change, we can stave off or even avoid intrusive conventional medical treatment and reduce the need for medications. A multidimensional approach to heart health greatly improves quality of life and helps return focus to the things that matter most in our lives.

chapter three

Heart Disease Risks

About eight out of 10 people have at least one risk factor for heart disease, while one in 10 has at least three or more. The more risk factors we have, the higher our risk of developing this progressive condition. Some risk factors, we are born with. Others, we develop – mostly from neglect or ignorance. Luckily, we can reduce our risk factors through diet, lifestyle, exercise, supplements and attention to stress and mental/emotional health.

Age
Aging inevitably puts us at higher risk of developing health issues. Our systems wear down. Heart function slows, and our arteries lose flexibility and fill with plaque. About 80 percent of people 65 and older have some form of heart disease. People of this age group also have a greater likelihood of having high blood pressure or diabetes. Compared to men, women's overall health by the time they are diagnosed with heart disease is worse, as is the progression of the disease itself.

Although heart disease tends to show up in adulthood, younger generations aren't immune to the processes that lead to this condition. Atherosclerosis can start as early as childhood. Rising rates of diabetes and obesity in kids and youths also put them at greater risk for future health problems. A team of US researchers recently did a statistical analysis to determine the potential impact of overweight adolescents on future adult heart health. They estimated that, by 2020, when the teens in their analysis turn 35, 37 percent of males and 44 percent of females will be obese, resulting in more heart attacks, chronic angina and deaths by the age of 50. They also estimated an additional 100,000 cases of heart disease by 2035, and up to a 19 percent increase in obesity-related coronary heart disease deaths. Clearly, if only from a cardiovascular perspective, it's critically important that we promote healthy eating and fitness principles to children at a young age and instill in them positive lifelong habits.

Gender

Heart disease is the leading cause of death in North America for both sexes. Until about age 40, men are more likely to suffer a heart-related event. After that, the tables turn and it's women who grow more at risk. Female hearts are smaller, the inner diameter of their arteries narrower, which makes the arteries more prone to blockage and damage. This sizing difference could also contribute to the higher heart attack mortality rates and increased risk of complications and death after bypass surgery and angioplasty in women.

■ *A Thyroid Connection*

Women are far more likely than men to have low thyroid function (hypothyroidism), which can worsen heart disease and its symptoms. The thyroid gland is important for metabolism, digestion, and muscle function. When the thyroid doesn't produce enough thyroid hormone, the heart can't contract and relax effectively, thus inhibiting its pumping strength. If unaddressed, diastolic dysfunction can occur, whereby the heart ventricles "stiffen," resulting in irregular blood flow and pooling. In serious cases, blood pools in the organs, mainly in the lungs, causing congestion and possible heart failure. Low thyroid function further increases C-reactive protein, a marker for inflammation, and is also very important in cholesterol metabolism.

People with severe hypothyroidism have higher elevated total and LDL cholesterol and, in 2003, the American Thyroid Association noted that even mild thyroid failure can elevate blood cholesterol.

Clinical hypothyroidism is diagnosed when your thyroid stimulating hormone (TSH) reading is higher than 5, but a TSH as low as 2 can cause low thyroid symptoms such as fatigue, weight gain, hair loss, irritability and dry, scaly skin. If you have low thyroid function or suspect that you do, have your hormone levels (re)checked. Most cases of thyroid dysfunction go undiagnosed. Symptoms related to the cardiac-thyroid connection include:

- A slow heart beat (thyroid modulates heart beat)
- Shortness of breath and inability to exercise (caused by weakened muscles)
- High diastolic blood pressure (due to stiffer arteries)
- Swelling (edema; often a symptom of heart failure)
- Worsening of heart failure
- Hastening of atherosclerosis.

♡ Heart Disease and HRT

Drug manufacturers of Premarin and Prempro (synthetic estrogens) have been told to put a strong warning on the label about the increased risk of cancer and heart disease. In July 2002, the Women's Health Initiative study, a clinical trial designed to determine if HRT, a combination of synthetic estrogen and progestins, was beneficial to healthy women. The study was halted due to serious safety concerns. This study involving 16,608 healthy, postmenopausal women concluded that the combination of estrogen and progestins caused a 41 percent increase in the risk of stroke, a 29 percent increase in the risk of heart attack, a doubled risk of blood clots, a 22 percent increase in cardiovascular disease and a 26 percent increase in the risk of invasive breast cancer.

In 2003, they discovered these drugs also doubled the risk of dementia, increased hearing loss and promoted asthma. In 2004, they stopped the estrogen only arm of the study due to an increased risk of stroke and dementia.

In January 2004, the Canadian Cancer Society sent out a strong warning about the cancer-causing effects of HRT. They stated, "Currently there are about five million women over the age of 50. Based on the results of the WHI study, if even 100,000 of those women take combined HRT for four years, we'll end up with an additional 80 cases of breast cancer." Up until the warning, the Canadian Cancer Society felt women should simply discuss HRT with their doctors, now they suggest women should avoid it. Maybe the warning is because too many doctors recommended women not worry about the negative news reports about HRT.

Much has been made of the heart-protective "estrogen" advantage that women have until menopause, when estrogen production declines. However, HRT is not the answer for heart disease prevention and, in fact, is damaging. Following a Heart-Smart lifestyle, eating well, exercising often, and supplementing wisely is side-effect-free and supports overall health far more than any synthetic pharmaceutical. For caring physicians and women are looking for alternatives to HRT due to menopausal symptoms, European doctors have been recommending herbal solutions for decades and the research is very clear they are safer and just as effective in 80 percent of users. Herbs and nutrients such as black cohosh, chasteberry (vitex) and dong quai, can halt hot flashes, night sweats and mood swings, lower cholesterol, improve vaginal dryness and more. For more information about herbs, foods and the use of bioidentical hormones, a safer option than synthetic HRT, read my book *A Smart Woman's Guide to Hormones*.

Family History

Although heart disease runs in families, this risk factor isn't as important as most people believe. A family history of heart disease increases the risk by only 25 percent. In context, this is roughly one-tenth as dangerous as smoking. So if your mother's second cousin has heart disease, you really needn't worry about this particular factor. The connection has to be quite close to qualify as a risk: a mother or sister before age 65, or a father or brother before 55. And even if you have a family history of heart disease, you *don't* have to eat like them.

Where genetics pale, familial behavior steps in. If your parents go heavy on meat and potatoes and drizzle them with gravy, you'll likely do the same. If you cook the same meals, you'll pass these habits on to your children. Similarly, unhealthy behaviors like smoking, drinking too much and dealing with stress poorly are often learned as well. So the question is, is it genetics or the transfer of unhealthy habits that creates the increased risk of heart disease amongst families?

Smoking

What can be said about smoking that you haven't already heard 100 times? Smoking causes heart harm by promoting atherosclerosis, reducing good HDL cholesterol and encouraging the formation of blood clots. Smokers die from heart disease more often – almost three times more often – than they die from lung cancer. They have double the risk of heart attack compared to non-smokers.

Women who smoke and take birth control pills experience more cardiac damage. Women who take high-estrogen birth control pills and smoke have a heart attack risk more than 35 times higher than a non-smoker. While a male smoker's risk of heart attack increases three-fold over non-smokers, female smokers have up to six times the risk of heart attack compared to non-smoking women.

Obesity

Being 20 percent higher than your ideal weight more than doubles your chance of developing heart disease. Your heart has to work harder for you to do even small tasks like crawl out of bed or lift a child onto your lap. Being overweight and obese is also associated with other heart disease risk factors, including high LDL cholesterol and blood pressure, and elevated triglycerides and blood sugar (glucose). The inflammation that plays a role in plaque formation in the arteries is also linked to our weight. A 1999 *Journal of the American Medical Association* study reported that obese people have higher levels of C-reactive protein, a marker for inflammation. In this study, obese men had levels of C-reactive protein five times higher than lean men, while women's levels were even higher. Obese women were 13 times more likely to have higher C-reactive protein levels than lean women.

> ♡ **Apples Versus Pears – A Weighty Issue**
>
> Heart speaking, an "apple" shape, where excess weight is carried in the upper body, is more dangerous than extra weight carried below the waist – the classic "pear" figure. Abdominal fat (love handles) breaks down easier into fatty acids that raise blood triglyceride levels. It also contributes to inflammation and insulin resistance, both of which have implications for heart disease.

One standard way to measure obesity is the body mass index (BMI). One advantage of this calculation is that it considers both weight and height. Calculate your percentage of body fat fairly accurately by cross-matching your figures on the following chart.

♡ Body Mass Index (BMI) Table

BMI	19	20	21	22	23	24	25	26	27	28	29	30	31	32	33	34	35
Height							*Weight (in Pounds)*										
4'10"	91	96	100	105	110	115	119	124	129	134	138	143	148	153	158	162	167
4'11"	94	99	104	109	114	119	124	128	133	138	143	148	153	158	163	168	173
5'	97	102	107	112	118	123	128	133	138	143	148	153	158	163	168	174	179
5'1"	100	106	111	116	122	127	132	137	143	148	153	158	164	169	174	180	185
5'2"	104	109	115	120	126	131	136	142	147	153	158	164	169	175	180	186	191
5'3"	107	113	118	124	130	135	141	146	152	158	163	169	175	180	186	191	197
5'4"	110	116	122	128	134	140	145	151	157	163	169	174	180	186	192	197	204
5'5"	114	120	126	132	138	144	150	156	162	168	174	180	186	192	198	204	210
5'6"	118	124	130	136	142	148	155	161	167	173	179	186	192	198	204	210	216
5'7"	121	127	134	140	146	153	159	166	172	178	185	191	198	204	211	217	223
5'8"	125	131	138	144	151	158	164	171	177	184	190	197	203	210	216	223	230
5'9"	128	135	142	149	155	162	169	176	182	189	196	203	209	216	223	230	236
5'10"	132	139	146	153	160	167	174	181	188	195	202	209	216	222	229	236	243
5'11"	136	143	150	157	165	172	179	186	193	200	208	215	222	229	236	243	250
6'	140	147	154	162	169	177	184	191	199	206	213	221	228	235	242	250	258
6'1"	144	151	159	166	174	182	189	197	204	212	219	227	235	242	250	257	265
6'2"	148	155	163	171	179	186	194	202	210	218	225	233	241	249	256	264	272
6'3"	152	160	168	176	184	192	200	208	216	224	232	240	248	256	264	272	279

A healthy BMI reading falls between 18.5 and 24, while anything above that puts us at an increased risk of heart disease. Twenty-five to 29 is overweight, while 30 or more is considered obese.

If you are a trained athlete, your weight based on a measured percentage of body fat would be a better indicator of what you should weigh. A normal healthy man shouldn't exceed 15 percent body fat, while the healthy limit for a woman is 15 to 22 percent.

Due to a few limitations with the BMI index, when considering body weight composition and associated health risks, experts often look at both BMI and our waist-to-hip ratio. Try the latter quick and dirty method of analysis yourself. You'll need a tape measure.

STEP ONE: With a tape measure, measure the circumference of your waist at its narrowest (usually around the navel). Be sure to relax your abdomen or your reading won't be accurate.

STEP TWO: Measure your hips at the widest point (usually around the large fleshy part of the buttocks).

STEP THREE: Divide your waist measurement by your hip measurement.

For women, a healthy waist-to-hip ratio is considered to be less than 0.8; for men, less than 0.9. With ratios above these, the risk of heart attack and stroke increases significantly in both sexes. Canadian researchers who studied 27,000 people from 52 countries reported in 2005 that men and women who'd had a heart attack had much higher waist-to-hip ratios than those who were heart-attack-free.

Inactivity
Overweight and inactivity go together like baked potatoes and sour cream. Lack of exercise contributes to weight gain and also puts added strain on your heart. Conversely, the positive effects of physical activity are well substantiated, and we know that even moderate activity can have heart-health effects. By improving vascular function, exercise strengthens the heart's performance. It also reduces adrenaline levels, improves muscular function, improves our blood lipid (fat) profile and reduces the risk of fatal arrhythmias. Studies show that exercise can significantly prolong the life expectancy of patients with heart failure.

In the *British Medical Journal* in 2004, data from nine clinical trials involving more than 800 heart failure patients showed that, irrespective of the underlying causes of heart failure, all patients in the exercise treatment group lived longer and had fewer hospital admissions. Similar results were reported in the *Journal of the American College of Cardiology* in 2006. Almost 100 patients received either conventional heart failure therapy alone or in combination with a nine-month aerobic exercise regimen. The exercise group had significantly lower levels of a hormone (BNP) known to occur with worsening heart failure and they had much improved cardiovascular function.

Above are just two of dozens of studies recognizing exercise's heart healthy effects. It's important to note that you don't have to be an Olympic athlete to achieve a positive effect; even a brisk half-hour walk daily that induces a light sweat, combined with regular weight training, can strengthen your cardiovascular system and chip away at excess calories. If necessary, please work with a fitness trainer or join a local community center program to help guide and motivate you.

♡ Calories Burned by Physical Activity

These are the calories expended by a 125 pound (57 kg) woman doing 10 minutes of the following activities.

ACTIVITY	CALORIES EXPENDED
Making beds	32
Weeding	49
Dancing	35
Swimming (front crawl)	40
Tennis	56
Walking (briskly)	52
Walking (leisurely stroll)	29
Running	90
Cycling	42
Cross-country skiing	98
Downhill skiing	80
Shoveling snow	65

chapter four

The Lowdown on Cholesterol and Blood Pressure

Cardiovascular disease is preventable and reversible if you follow a Heart-Smart lifestyle. High cholesterol and high blood pressure are just two risk factors that respond amazingly well to diet, exercise, nutritional supplements and anti-stress strategies.

High Cholesterol

As was pointed out earlier, there are few substances as controversial as cholesterol, and no substance about which there is more confusion. We need cholesterol, yet it can also play an undesirable role in atherosclerosis. When small injuries or nicks occur in the arteries, cholesterol, which acts as an internal Band-Aid, can get out of control and, with the help of other factors, clog arteries and increase our risk of heart attack and heart damage.

"Bad" LDL cholesterol contributes to heart disease. But it can be kept in line by "good" HDL cholesterol, which helps to sweep LDL through the body and also helps to prevent LDL from oxidizing. Oxidized LDL causes plaque formation, inflammation and damage to neighbouring cells. As if this weren't enough, there are very low density lipoproteins (VLDL) to watch out for. These extra small bad cholesterol particles are more likely to both form arterial plaques and oxidize due to free radical damage. People with lots of smaller LDL particles have a higher risk of heart disease than those with larger LDL particles.

Cholesterol Levels		
	US (mg/dL)	Canada (mmol/L)
Total Cholesterol		
Ideal	<200	<5.2
Borderline high	201-239	5.2-6.1
High	>240	>6.2
LDL Cholesterol		
Ideal	<100	<2.6
Middle range	100-159	2.7-4.1
High	160-189	4.2-4.9
Very high	>190	>4.9/5.0
HDL Cholesterol		
Low	<40	<1.0
High	>60	>1.6

About 40 percent of North Americans have higher than recommended cholesterol levels, although it's important to keep in mind that "recommendations" continue to evolve along with our understanding of the mechanisms behind heart disease. Traditionally, it was believed that your total cholesterol measure (derived by adding LDL and HDL levels together) was the best predictor of heart disease risk. It's now held that the ratio of total-to-HDL cholesterol is more accurate. For people with zero or one risk factor for developing heart disease in the next 10 years, a ratio of 6:1 is considered acceptable. However, if you are at moderate or higher risk of developing heart disease with two or more risk factors – the category into which most people fall – maintaining a lower ratio through diet, lifestyle, supplements and fitness is very important. Generally, the lower the ratio, the better, with an ideal ratio being about 4:1.

The traditional cholesterol test used for decades gives readings for LDL, HDL and triglycerides, but not for newer heart disease indicators. You may require a specialized test requisitioned through your health-care provider. The newer VAP cholesterol test is very comprehensive and likely to catch on in medical testing circles although it is still relatively unused in North America. The VAP test categorizes LDL cholesterol by size, identifies HDL subclasses (some of which are more heart-protective than others), measures very low density lipoprotein (VLDL), and more. It's valuable to know your VLDL reading as another marker in your lipid (fat) profile. A "normal" VLDL reading is 5-40 mg/dL (0.1-1.0 mmol/L).

Good Cholesterol
Let's look further at "good" HDL cholesterol. HDL is particularly relevant to women. For women, having low HDL is even more of a risk factor than having high "bad" LDL. Even small decreases in HDL cholesterol after menopause significantly increases the risk of heart disease. In fact, HDL cholesterol is so protective that a low amount is considered an independent risk factor for heart disease.

HDL Cholesterol Ranges		
		Increased risk
Females, to age 19	0.9-2.4 mmol/L (CAN) 35-93 mg/dL (US)	<0.9 mmol/L (CAN) <35 mg/dL (US)
Females, 20+	>1.3 mmol/L (CAN) >50 mg/dL (US)	<1.3 mmol/L (CAN) <50 mg/dL (US)

Males to age 19	0.9-1.6 mmol/L (CAN)	<0.9 mmol/L (CAN)
	35-62 mg/dL (US)	<35 mg/dL (US)
Males, 20+	>1.0 mmol/L (CAN)	<1.0 mmol/L (CAN)
	>39 mg/dL (US)	<39 mg/dL (US)

Maintaining a healthy cholesterol profile is very achievable. Nine out of 10 people can lower high LDL, lower VLDL and improve HDL with dietary changes and nutritional supplements alone. Only 10 percent of people will require medication to keep levels in check. This is probably a shock to most people, considering that cholesterol-lowering statins are the number one prescribed drug in North America and that every time official "recommended" cholesterol levels drop (as they have several times), millions more North Americans are encouraged to take pharmaceuticals to lower LDL. This raises a point to consider. How low is too low when it comes to LDL? Some research indicates that it may serve more of a physiological purpose than previously thought. Researchers reported in the *Canadian Medical Association Journal* in 2008 that "LDL cholesterol levels below 2.8 mmol/L [108 mg/dL] and levels of at least 3.9 mmol/L [150.9 mg/dL] were both associated with a markedly elevated risk of cancer." This study examined type 2 diabetics, who are prime consumers of statin-lowering drugs due to the link between diabetes and heart disease.

Another fact pointing to the need to question current cholesterol assumptions is that many heart attack victims have "normal" cholesterol levels. This has been noted in numerous studies, including, most recently, a 2009 study that looked at almost 137,000 Americans hospitalized for heart attacks between 2000 and 2006. Seventy-two percent had cholesterol levels suggesting that they were not at risk for cardiovascular disease. Clearly, cholesterol isn't the universal bad guy, and although cholesterol is a factor in heart health, it is not the only factor and should be considered as part of a complete cardiovascular health assessment.

Triglycerides

Like cholesterol, triglycerides are a blood fat. They're the most common form in the body and are manufactured in the liver. When we eat too many high-calorie, high-sugar foods (or drinks), and our body can't burn the energy off fast enough, blood triglyceride levels shoot up and we store them as fat. (Grab that extra roll around your middle and you're grabbing triglycerides.) Triglycerides slide through the bloodstream on the very low-density lipoproteins (VLDL) cholesterol particles that we have noted contribute to atherosclerosis and instigate free radical damage in the arteries.

Elevated triglyceride levels increase your risk of heart disease and are linked to diabetes and prediabetic syndromes such as syndrome X. Insulin resistance, which underlies all these metabolic conditions, essentially prompts the liver to produce more VLDL, which raises triglyceride levels. Our fatty blood grows sluggish and its ability to carry oxygen is reduced.

	Triglycerides (US)	Triglycerides (CAN)
Desirable	<150 mg/dL	<1.7 mmol/L
Borderline high	150-199 mg/dL	1.7-2.2 mmol/L
High	200-499 mg/dL	2.3-5.6 mmol/L
Very high	500 mg/dL and above	Above 5.6 mmol/L

Fortunately, also like cholesterol, triglycerides are very responsive to diet and lifestyle modifications and the nutritional supplements starting on page 51.

Lipoprotein(a) and Apolipoprotein B

Lipoprotein(a), Lp(a), is a type of LDL cholesterol that is indicated in increased heart disease risk. One British review in 2000 of 27 studies found that patients with elevated Lp(a) had a 70 percent increased risk of heart disease. Lp(a) is thought to hinder the ability to dissolve blood clots, thus increasing heart attack risk. Lp(a) also plays an inflammatory role in atherosclerosis and detrimentally affects the thickness and responsiveness of arteries.

Apolipoprotein B (Apo B) is found in the VLDL and LDL particles that cart cholesterol through your blood. This small, dense protein binds with receptors on the body's cells, promoting your uptake of cholesterol. Knowing your reading can help determine the type and/or cause of your high cholesterol. Even though there's a current lack of consensus about Apo B as an indicator of heart disease, it should be checked.

Testing for Lp(a) and Apo B is less common but still available through blood work requisitioned by your doctor. If you are deemed "at risk" for cardiovascular disease, it may be covered by extended medical or Canadian Medicare. The VAP test can also detect them, although VAP testing, if you can find a health-care provider who will arrange it, will likely be an out-of-pocket expense.

Normal values for Lp(a) are less than 30 mg/dL in the US and 0.8 mmol/L in Canada. For Apo B, the normal level is 40-125 mg/dL and a recommended 0.9 g/L respectively.

Homocysteine: Too Much of A Good Thing

To build and repair tissues and muscles, the body uses methionine, a protein. A byproduct of this process is the amino acid homocysteine. This is a normal inner function; however, unnaturally elevated levels of homocysteine in the blood damage the endothelium cells in the arteries and promote atherosclerosis. Homocysteine also stimulates abnormal growth of smooth muscle in the middle layer of the arteries, which can then thicken the wall and clog the artery in question. Homocysteine can also promote blood clots by stimulating the body's clotting mechanisms.

Elevated homocysteine triples the risk of heart attack, even after all other risk factors are accounted for, according to a 1992 study which monitored the health of a large group of physicians. In 1997, the *Journal of the American Medical Association* reported that a high total homocysteine level represents an independent risk factor for heart disease similar to that of smoking or high blood fats (cholesterols, triglycerides). It also powerfully increases the risk associated with smoking and high blood pressure. Fortunately, the body has a built-in mechanism for dealing with too much homocysteine. We need adequate amounts of folic acid and vitamins B6 and B12 to support methylation, which converts homocysteine into harmless elements. People who are deficient in these nutrients have high homocysteine levels. We can achieve adequate levels of B vitamins through a proper diet and by taking B vitamins, thus supporting homocysteine reduction pathways and reducing our risk of heart attack.

There is no universal "normal" or "safe" range of homocysteine. You will hear doctors say 5-15 mmol/L is standard. Most people are about 10 mmol/L, which is also the therapeutic target recommended by the American Heart Association. A typical cardiovascular risk profile ordered through a naturopathic doctor sets the range at 3-14 mmol/L. Any reading above 6.3 mmol/L is associated with a steep increase in heart attack risk so the lower end of the scale is a better target to aim for.

High Iron is Dangerous
Iron is needed for hemoglobin, a protein in the red blood cells that deliver oxygen throughout the body. We also need iron for energy, muscle tone and healthy organ function. While many people, especially vegetarians and the elderly, are at risk for iron deficiency, too much iron is an important marker of cardiovascular

health. Ischemic heart disease, iron overload and hemochromatosis (an inherited disorder where the body can't store iron properly) are associated with high levels of ferritin, a protein in cells that stores iron so the body can use it later.

A ferritin test indirectly assesses how much iron is stored in the body. The normal serum (blood) ranges are:
• Men: 12-300 nanograms per milliliter (ng/mL)
• Women: 12-150 ng/mL

The lower the reading, the greater the likelihood of iron deficiency. Symptoms include fatigue, weakness, lack of stamina, poor concentration, headache, pallor, irritability and a craving for ice.

Fibrinogen: Blood Clot Indicator
Without the blood's ability to stop bleeding, even the smallest cut or scrape would be life-threatening. When a blood vessel breaks, chemical messengers and clotting factors hurry to plug the injury, then convert the liquid in the vicinity into a thicker clotty gel. One of these clotting factors is fibrinogen, produced by the liver.

High levels of fibrinogen put us at increased risk for blood clots and, ultimately, for heart attack (as most heart attacks are caused by blood clots that form in arteries clogged by atherosclerotic plaque). A blood clot can also break away and travel via the bloodstream to lodge elsewhere. Following a heart attack, excess fibrinogen is a marker for increased mortality, according to a 2005 Italian study that followed 92 men for 42 months after they suffered a heart attack. After taking into account all other factors such as age, body mass index, blood pressure smoking and blood lipids (fats), fibrinogen levels were the only independent predictor of death. It has also been shown to be an independent marker for overall and cardiovascular mortality in patients with end-stage kidney disease, and as a marker for the silent brain vessel lesions that increase stroke risk. A large

2005 meta-analysis reported in the *Journal of the American Medical Association* noted "moderately strong" associations between usual plasma fibrinogen level and the risks of coronary heart disease, stroke and other vascular mortality.

Fibrinogen tests can be ordered by your doctor, or purchased online through various direct-to-consumer companies. According to the US National Institutes of Health, a "normal" fibrinogen range is 200-400 milligrams per deciliter (mg/dL) of blood. The Life Extension Foundation suggests optimal fibrinogen levels are between 215-300 mg/dL. The ranges on a typical naturopathic cardiovascular test profile are 175-425 mg/dL. Your reading should be considered within the context of your complete cardiovascular assessment profile. It is possible to reduce elevated fibrinogen by following the recommendations in the following chapters.

C-reactive Protein: Inflammation Agent
Have you ever sprained your finger or stubbed your toe? In response to injury, allergy or infection, the immune system snaps into action. White blood cells and other factors are discharged to facilitate healing, causing redness, pain and heat – all signs of inflammation.

Inflammation is a major factor in heart disease and the suspected reason why a surprisingly high percentage of people who have had a heart attack have normal cholesterol and blood pressure. Even in people with normal blood cholesterol, occasionally cholesterol finds its way into the lining of the arteries and is embedded there as plaque. (Those with high blood cholesterol are at greater risk of this happening.) Our immune response causes inflammation that triggers the eruption of these plaques and the formation of blood clots that silently set the stage for heart attacks.

C-reactive protein (CRP) is produced by the liver during an inflammatory response. In a large-scale Harvard study involving 540 physicians, men with the highest CRP levels were three times more likely to have a heart attack and twice as likely to have had a stroke than men with the lowest levels. One year later, in 1998, a study looked at C-reactive protein in women. This inflammatory marker beat out cholesterol levels as a predictor of heart attack or stroke. "Women who developed cardiovascular events had higher baseline CRP levels than control subjects... Those with the highest levels [ ] had a five-fold increase in risk of any vascular event and a seven-fold increase in risk of [heart attack] or stroke," the researchers reported. Women on HRT have to be particularly careful because estrogen (Premarin) increases inflammation in the body and elevates CRP to dangerous levels, including a much higher risk of heart attack and strokes.

♡ An Infection Connection

Certain micro-organisms tend to show up in atherosclerotic plaques and promote inflammation. One of these, *Chlamydia pneumoniae*, is a bacterium linked to gum disease, pneumonia, bronchitis and sinus infections. People with advanced gum disease are more likely to have heart disease, advanced atherosclerosis, and have an increased risk of stroke compared to people with healthy gums. The common herpes simplex virus type 1 is also thought to be a possible instigator/contributor to heart disease.

Endocarditis is a heart infection caused by bacteria invading the inner lining of the heart (endocardium). The heart valves are typically involved as well; a diseased or an artificial valve can invite bacteria to lodge on the surface and nest. This can also occur during procedures in dentistry and gut examination (e.g. colonoscopy). Symptoms include a low-grade fever, fatigue, and loss of appetite and weight. Endocarditis is usually treated by antibiotics and is quite serious, with a death rate of 20 percent.

The amount of CRP in the blood is a good indicator of how much inflammation is occurring anywhere in the body, including in the arteries. Ask your physician for a high-sensitivity CRP blood test. If you have a CRP level over 3.0 mg/L, you should work to locate the source of inflammation in the body and treat it quickly.

- Optimal: 0.5-1 mg/L
- Should be monitored: 1.0-3.0 mg/L
- Indicates high levels of inflammation: >3.0 mg/L

♡ Cardiovascular Health Profile Assessment		
TEST	**US UNITS**	**CANADIAN UNITS**
Total cholesterol	<200 mg/dL	<5.2 mmol/L
LDL cholesterol	<100 mg/dL	<2.6 mmol/L
HDL cholesterol		
• Men	>39 mg/dL	>1.0 mmol/L
• Women	>60 mg/dL	>1.6 mmol/L
Total-to-HDL cholesterol ratio for both countries 3:1		
VLDL cholesterol	5-40 mg/dl	0.1-1.0 mmol/L
Triglycerides	<150 mg/dL	<1.7 mmol/L
Lp(a)	<30 mg/dL	<0.8 mmol/L
Apo B	40-125 mg/dL	0.9 g/L
Homocysteine	6.3 mmol/L	6.3 mmol/L
Ferritin		
• Men	12-300 ng/mL	12-300 ng/mL
• Women	12–150 ng/mL	12–150 ng/mL
Fibrinogen	215-300 mg/dL	215-300 mg/dL
C-reactive protein	<1 mg/L	<1 mg/L

High Blood Pressure (Hypertension)

Imagine trying to squeeze dishwashing liquid through a bottle head that has become caked and blocked with solidified soap. You have to press harder to get any out, and when it does, it shoots out erratically.

A similar disturbance occurs in the one in three Americans and one in five Canadians who has high blood pressure, or hypertension. With this common condition, the heart muscle contracts too forcefully and sends blood driving through the body with excess strength. Clogged arteries can create additional resistance that causes damage in the sensitive inner endothelium layer. This "wear and tear" promotes the plaque buildup that leads to heart disease. People with high blood pressure are more than twice as likely to have a heart attack compared to people with normal blood pressure. Hypertension also strains and eventually weakens the heart, while very high blood pressure can cause blood vessels to burst in the brain, causing a stroke.

♡ Causes of High Blood Pressure

- Age (blood pressure generally increases with age)
- A poor diet
- Magnesium deficiency
- Too much alcohol
- Lack of exercise
- Obesity
- Stress
- Another health condition, e.g. kidney disease or thyroid dysfunction (both more common in women than men)
- Pregnancy
- Birth control pills
- Certain drugs, e.g. amphetamines (stimulants), diet pills and some cold and allergy pills

---

Systolic Versus Diastolic

A blood pressure reading has two parts, systolic pressure (the top number) and diastolic pressure (the bottom number). The higher systolic reading represents the pressure just after your heart beats (i.e. when your heart contracts and pushes blood out into arteries).

The lower diastolic reading is the pressure while your heart is at rest, refilling with blood between beats.

The ideal adult blood pressure reading is less than 120/80, measured in millimeters of mercury (mmHg). High blood pressure is considered anything higher than 140/90.

BLOOD PRESSURE	OPTIMAL	NORMAL	HIGH NORMAL	HYPERTENSION
Systolic	Less than 120	Less than 130	130-139	140 or higher
Diastolic	Less than 80	Less than 85	85-89	90 or higher

A new category of high blood pressure called "prehypertension" is between 130-139/85-89 mmHg. Sixty percent of people with prehypertension will graduate to hypertension within four years unless they make heart-healthy diet, fitness, and lifestyle changes designed to bring their blood pressure back down. Even a 1 mmHg drop in diastolic blood pressure can shrink your risk for heart disease by two to three percent.

Have your blood pressure checked regularly. Because high blood pressure generally doesn't cause overt symptoms, one-fifth of Americans and two-fifths of Canadians don't know they have it. Like heart disease, blood pressure abnormalities respond well to non-invasive, non-medicated methods of intervention.

chapter five

Diabetes and Depression: Double Trouble

Imagine two foods on a table in front of you. The first is a hardboiled egg, the second a white cupcake with chocolate icing. How would these foods be metabolized in your body? The protein-rich egg would slowly and steadily be digested without a spike in glucose (blood sugar). The pancreas would be triggered to produce normal amounts of insulin to assist glucose uptake into the cells. That cellular uptake would be equally gradual, and you would experience an even energy level until the next influx of food, hopefully an equally healthy choice.

Since glucose is the main fuel for our brain, it's important to balance our blood sugar in a way that supplies the body's demands. But, ahhh, that cupcake is tempting. And imagine what happens when you eat it. The refined flour, void of fiber and nutrients, is used by the body in the same way as pure sugar. It hits the bloodstream quickly, demanding an influx of insulin from the pancreas, which pumps out the hormone needed to shuttle glucose into cells. The cells take a huge sugar hit, resulting in a "sugar high" that leaves you buzzing. But before you know it, that quick burst of energy is gone. You're exhausted yet left craving the next sugary sweet.

Steady Sugar Destruction

The cumulative effect of unhealthy food choices is destructive. If you indulge in a steady supply of high-sugar and/or high-carbohydrate processed foods, your body systems are going to become overwhelmed. Your pancreas can get overworked and will stop producing the insulin you need. Or maybe your cells become less inclined to heed insulin's call and slow the uptake of glucose, otherwise known as insulin resistance. One third of North Americans have some form of insulin resistance in which your fasting glucose level (the amount of sugar in your bloodstream after several hours of no food or drink) is higher than normal but not high enough for a diabetes diagnosis. Over time, if you don't address this dangerous precursor, your blood sugar and insulin will continue to rise and a type 2 diabetes diagnosis will result.

Type 1 diabetes accounts for 10 percent of cases and usually begins during childhood. In type 1 diabetics, the immune system has destroyed the beta cells of the pancreas that produce insulin, so daily insulin injections are required. Nine out of 10 cases of diabetes are of the type 2 variety, which usually starts around age 40 – in other words, around the time that inactivity and the effects of the typical North American diet catches up with us. Our pancreas and cells shout out, "No more terrible diet and lifestyle choices!" Our heart gratefully echoes the sentiment. According to the American Diabetes Association, two out of every three people with diabetes dies of some form of heart or blood vessel disease.

Not Sweet for the Heart

It is misleading to focus solely on the "diabetic" effect on the heart. It would be more accurate to refer to the heart disease risks caused by all prediabetic states including insulin resistance, in which blood glucose levels are unnaturally high. According to a 2001 *British Medical Journal* study, even elevated blood glucose is a powerful predictor of heart disease.

Excess sugar in the blood damages blood vessels by contributing to the fat deposits on their walls, which leads to atherosclerosis, blocked arteries and all too often to heart attacks and heart damage. Too much sugar also makes blood thicker and stickier, hindering the blood's ability to deliver nutrients and oxygen to the cells. Circulation and blood flow slows – not a good thing considering how much energy and oxygen the heart needs to sustain its pumping effects.

When we have too much glucose in the blood, it triggers the liver to make more very low density lipoproteins (VLDL) that carry triglycerides in the blood and also cause free radical damage. Consequently, diabetes and other irregular blood sugar syndromes contribute to high triglycerides and increase bad cholesterol. At the same time, the amount of good HDL cholesterol in the body decreases. This combination of high triglycerides, high bad cholesterol and low good cholesterol puts us at risk for heart disease. The inflammation brigade also wants in on the action. Persistent irregular sugar regulation increases fibrinogen and C-reactive protein, higher levels of which increase artery clogging and heart attack.

Sugar Speeds Aging
Yet another biochemical process related to (pre)diabetic states and heart disease – as well as premature aging – is glycation. When blood sugar binds to and chemically alters proteins and fats, damage occurs. These damaged molecules are called advanced glycation end products and they interfere with the way cells work. They bind with collagen and make blood vessels stiff. They also promote blood clots by attracting blood platelets, encourage the oxidation of LDL cholesterol and create low-grade inflammation that promotes atherosclerosis.

Lifestyle Is the Best Drug
If you are even 15-20 pounds overweight, you could be at risk for diabetes and heart disease. Have a glucose tolerance test to

determine how quickly glucose is cleared from your blood. "Normal" blood values for the 75-gram oral glucose tolerance test that is used to check for type 2 diabetes are:
- Fasting: 60-100 mg/dL
- 1 hour: <200 mg/dL
- 2 hours: <140 mg/dL. Between 140-200 mg/dL is considered impaired glucose tolerance (or prediabetes, when the body has become less sensitive to insulin and has to work harder to control blood glucose levels). This group is at increased risk for developing diabetes. Greater than 200 mg/dL is a sign of type 2 diabetes.

Sometimes, blood sugar problems that generate readings too low to be diagnosed by traditional tests go unaddressed and cause a variety of seemingly unrelated symptoms, including anxiety, fatigue, irritability and poor concentration. Tested or untested, everybody can benefit by working to keep blood sugars balanced and controlling the processes that create diabetes and long-term complications such as kidney, eye and nerve damage.

Diabetes Prevention
In one compelling study on diabetes prevention, 3,200 non-diabetics with elevated blood sugar readings were placed into three groups: one taking a placebo, one taking a common insulin drug, and one with a lifestyle-modification program including two-and-a-half hours of exercise per week. After three years, diabetes incidence was 11 cases per 100 people in the placebo group, eight per 100 in the drug group and five per 100 in the lifestyle/exercise group. In other words, while drug therapy was more effective than placebo at preventing diabetes, a change in lifestyle was the most effective. Diet and exercise intervention reduced the incidence of diabetes by 58 percent. Similar findings about lifestyle and exercise's effect on diabetes prevention have been repeated since.

A recent study confirms that by taking steps to regulate blood sugar metabolism, we can also help stop heart disease in its tracks. More than 3,000 participants with impaired glucose tolerance were separated into three groups: one placebo group, one taking a common insulin drug, and one that underwent lifestyle modifications including a calorie-restricted diet and moderate exercise. Over three years, tests were conducted to assess blood sugar changes and trends in risk factors for cardiovascular disease, including blood pressure, triglycerides and cholesterol levels. The researchers found that as glucose tolerance status deteriorated, cardiovascular risk factors went downhill as well. Conversely, when blood sugar regulation improved, the risk factors improved. The researchers concluded that changing your lifestyle is more effective than taking an insulin drug at improving your glucose tolerance profile *and* cardiovascular risk.

Clearly, heart disease and diabetes (and prediabetic states) are largely diseases created by poor choices. Let's attack two killers with the power of a healthy, active lifestyle, supported by a low-glycemic diet, regular stress-reducing activities and good mental/emotional health practices.

Heart Disease Linked to Depression

Whether we're taking preventive steps, whether we've suffered a heart attack, or whether we've had surgery, our emotions and mental state play a huge role in heart health.

Depression sufferers are four times more likely to develop heart disease. Some suggest this because people with depressive personalities are more likely to engage in destructive habits like smoking, drinking and overeating, and are less likely to regularly exercise or embrace stress reduction and healing mind-body strategies. Others favor biochemical explanations because there is a definite connection between what's going on inside our hearts, and external psychosocial factors such as how we think, feel and react to the (lack of) people around us.

Women More At Risk

Research shows that women are more vulnerable to depression than men. About twice as many women suffer from this affliction, a statistic echoed in most countries around the world regardless of our ethnic, racial and economic situations. A combination of uniquely feminine factors put women more at risk. Biologically, female hormones are intricately entwined with their emotions.

Menstruation, pregnancy, postpartum "baby blues," perimenopause and menopause – these are just a few specific situations in a woman's life when hormonal chemical messengers can cause major mood fluctuations. Socially and culturally, women are under strain from the multiple roles they play (wife, mother, career woman), while low income puts women more at risk of depression.

♡ Symptoms of Depression

- No interest or pleasure in things you used to enjoy
- Feeling sad or empty
- Crying easily or unexplained crying
- Feeling slowed down or restless
- Feeling worthless or guilty
- Change in appetite leading to weight gain or loss
- Thinking about death or suicide
- Concentration or memory troubles
- Trouble making everyday decisions
- Problems sleeping, especially in the early morning, or wanting to sleep all of the time or "hide under the covers"
- Feeling tired all of the time
- Feeling numb emotionally, perhaps even to the point of not being able to cry

If you think depression is affecting you, sharing this concern with a trusted professional is important. Many people with depression aren't adequately treated, and, in women, depression is misdiagnosed 30 to 50 percent of the time.

Achy, Breaky Heart

When we are depressed, the nervous system is stimulated and puts stress on the heart. Heart rate and blood pressure increase and the risk of an irregular heartbeat (arrhythmia) rises. Depression causes dysfunction of our "happy hormone" serotonin, which encourages blood platelets to clump together, creating blood clots that can eventually clog arteries and cause heart attacks.

People with depression have more heart attacks and are more likely to die of sudden death. In one study of 2,800 heart-disease-free participants, those suffering from major depression were three times more likely to develop fatal heart disease within four years than those who weren't depressed. A 2009 study in *Journal of the American College of Cardiology* confirmed this link, evaluating 63,000 women from the long-running Nurses Health Study (1992-2004). None had heart disease signs at the study's beginning; eight percent showed signs of serious depression. The depressed women were over twice as likely to die from sudden cardiac death, frequently caused by arrhythmia. They were also slightly more likely to die from coronary heart disease than the women without depression.

Formulate Your Heart-health Plan

Not only is depression a heart disease "precursor", but people who have a cardiac event (e.g. a heart attack) or who are in recovery mode (after a surgery) are also prone to depression, which actually increases the chance of another heart attack and/or heart-disease-related fatality. Another recent study in the journal *Circulation* also suggests that depression further increases the risk of atherosclerotic progression.

After a heart attack or surgery, it's crucially important to formulate a heart-health plan. Gather a supportive team comprised of health-care advisors and family, friends, club members, someone from your religious faith – whoever you think you need. If depression is a part of your life, or if you think you might be depressed, your team may involve a counselor or psychologist – again, someone you feel comfortable with to help guide you to better mental and emotional health.

Lifesaving Support
Friends and family keep us healthy. People with healthier support networks report better health. Single people have higher death rates than married people. Retired men, men who have often given up a huge portion of their lifelong identity – their work – have almost double the risk of suffering from a fatal heart attack than employed men. Men and women with poor social support are more likely to suffer complications during cardiovascular surgery. In early 1980s research, Hawaiian men with large social networks (family, work, church, social groups) were less likely to suffer a heart attack, angina or other form of heart disease. Interestingly, the stronger a man's social connections, the lesser the risk. In 2003, in a review of that evidence, National Heart Foundation of Australia researchers concluded in the *Medical Journal of Australia* that "there is strong and consistent evidence of an independent causal association between depression, social isolation and lack of quality social support and the causes and prognosis of coronary heart disease."

♡ **Pets Invited**

Animals are very heart-healthy. In the aftermath of a heart attack, dog owners are significantly more likely to be alive one year later, regardless of how severe the attack was, according to a National Institutes of Health study involving 421 adults. In another study involving 240 married couples, those with pets had lower blood pressure and heart rates in times of both relaxation and stress, compared to non-pet owners.

Owning a dog also invites more opportunities to get out there and walk, as other studies have shown. Dog owners get more exercise, resulting in other heart benefits and greater mobility.

Anger Hurts the Heart

In times of anger and heightened emotions, numerous physical changes are activated. We tense up as if preparing for battle. Cortisol, a "stress" hormone, surges through our system. Our heartbeat speeds up and our arteries constrict, raising blood pressure, triglycerides and cholesterol. Simultaneously, our heart's need for oxygen to sustain these changes increases. This set of factors is why angina (chest pain) is a common symptom during bouts of anger and panic attacks. Stress, cortisol and other hormones, meanwhile, are also getting busy elsewhere in the body (see page 103).

People prone to anger, hostility and cynicism are especially vulnerable to heart disease. Living in this state of chronically elevated stress hormones sets the stage for high blood pressure, arterial damage and atherosclerosis. In one Harvard study of 1,600 participants who'd had a heart attack, eight percent reported being angry in the 24 hours prior to the attack. Those who also reported intense anger in the two hours prior had double the heart attack risk. In 2009, researchers did a meta-analysis of 44 studies on coronary heart disease and anger and hostility. These emotions, they concluded, impact heart disease outcomes in both healthy populations and in people with existing heart disease. In other words, whether we have heart disease or want to avoid it, learning to appropriately handle our emotions is essential.

♡ Anxiety – The False Heart Attack

Poor Jack Nicholson's character in the film *Something's Gotta Give*. You can't help but feel bad for him as he suffers what he thinks is a heart attack after being rejected by Diane Keaton's character, only to later be told by a doctor (Keanu Reeves) that he'd had a panic attack instead.

Heart attacks and anxiety attacks have overlapping symptoms so it's easy to understand where the mistake was made. Both involve an increased heart rate and an irregular beat, and both are painful and uncomfortable. With a heart attack, however, the severity of pain is usually stronger and may affect other parts of the upper body besides the chest – the arms, jaw, neck, stomach (for other heart attack (sex-specific) symptoms, see page 11).

Heart attack victims don't tend to hyperventilate, while people having a panic attack might (unless it was the panic attack that triggered the heart attack). Through learned techniques, such as deep breathing and relaxation exercises, panic attacks can be controlled and heart disease progression leading to heart attack alleviated.

Gone are the days when heart disease was considered strictly a physical phenomena, the mind and body disassociated from each other. Thinking on this point has come full circle in the past few decades, supported by a growing body of research. Simply put, heal our minds, heal our emotions, heal our hearts.

chapter six

Heart-Smart Personal Assessment

Circle your responses, then tally up the corresponding points and read about your heart disease risk assessment on page 50.

I'm...

Male	0
Female	1

I'm...

Less than 30 years old	0
30-50 years old	1
More than 50 years old	2

My total cholesterol is...

Less than 5.2 mmol/L (200 mg/dL)	0
5.3-6.1 mmol/L (200-239 mg/dL)	1
Greater than 6.2 mmol/L (240 mg/dL)	2

For a woman: My HDL cholesterol is...

Greater than 1.3 mmol/L (50 mg/dL)	0
Less than 1.3 mmol/L (50 mg/dL)	1

For a man: My HDL cholesterol is...

Greater than 1.0 mmol/L (39 mg/dL)	0
Less than 1.0 mmol/L (39 mg/dL)	1

My triglycerides are...

Less than 1.7 mmol/L (150 mg/dL)	0
1.7-2.2 mmol/L (150-199 mg/dL)	1
2.3-5.6 mmol/L (200-499 mg/dL)	2

My lipoprotein(a) is...

Less than 0.8 mmol/L (30 mg/dL)	0
Greater than 0.8 mmol/L (30 mg/dL)	1

My homocysteine is...

Less than 6.3 mmol/L	0
Greater than 6.3 mmol/L	1

My C-reactive protein is...

Less than 1 mg/L	0
1-3 mg/L	1
Greater than 3 mg/L	2

My blood pressure is...

120/80 to 130/85 mmHg	0
130-139/85-89 mmHg	1
140/90 mmHg or higher	2

I have a family history of heart disease
(i.e. a mother or sister before age 55, or a father or brother before 65).

No	0
Yes	1

I smoke.

No	0
Yes	2

My body mass index (BMI) is...

18.5-24	0
25-29	1
30 or higher	2

My body shape is that of...

A pear	0
An apple	1

I have...

diabetes	2
irregular blood sugar metabolism	1
regular blood sugar metabolism	0

I...

Have depression	2
Have previously been diagnosed with depression	1
Have never suffered from depression	0

I exercise _____ a week, including activities such as brisk walking, swimming, biking, dancing and active gardening.

4 or more times	0
2-3 times	1
0-1	2

I would rate my social support system as...

Good	0
Fair	1
Poor	2

My main sources of protein are...

Red meats	2
Chicken and other poultry	1
Seafood and fish	0

I eat mostly _____ daily.

Trans fats (fried/processed foods)	2
Saturated fats (animal fats/processed foods)	1
Unprocessed and unsaturated fats and oils (of largely vegetarian origin)	0

My carbohydrate choices are...

Mostly high glycemic items	2
Mostly medium glycemic items	1
Mostly low glycemic items	0

I eat a lot of canned foods and often add salt to my diet.	2
I don't watch my salt intake.	1
I watch my salt intake and try to avoid excess salt.	0

I drink more than 9 drinks a week (for women) or 14 drinks a week (for men).

Yes.	1
No.	0

In a typical week, I feel stressed...

Almost every day	2
A few times	1
Rarely	0

Your Heart-Smart Score

30-39: High risk.
It's long past time to start reducing your risk by making diet and lifestyle changes. Find out how in the following chapters.

20-29: Moderate/high risk.
Your heart needs help. Let's ramp up your heart-healthy efforts from medium to high speed.

10-19: Low/medium risk.
Not bad at all, but there is room for improvement.

0-9: Low risk.
Congratulations on your current heart smarts! Follow the Heart-Smart Program to keep yourself on track.

chapter seven

The Heart-Smart Diet

Several times a day, we have a chance to make decisions that can, quite literally, save our lives. If we choose 14-ounce steaks and French fries, skip the salad and gorge on ice cream, we're also clogging our system with unhealthy fats and promoting "bad" LDL cholesterol buildup and atherosclerosis. We're forcing our heart (and other organs) to work harder, increasing underlying inflammation and other markers for heart disease and... the list goes on.

What Is a Carbohydrate?

The three main components of food are protein, carbohydrates (carbs) and fats, and all are used for fuel in the body. Although protein and fats are the main sources of fuel used for repair, maintenance and growth of all cells in the body, in our modern day diet, we tend to eat far too many carbohydrates. When carbs are present in abundance, our bodies convert them to fat.

Carbohydrates supply us with energy. The body converts all carbohydrates, with the exception of fiber, into glucose (blood sugar). Found predominantly in plant foods and, to a lesser extent, in milk and milk products, carbohydrates are divided into two groups: complex carbohydrates, which are made up of hundreds of sugar molecules linked together, and simple carbohydrates, which usually contain up to three sugar molecules. Simple carbohydrates are often sweet and are found in refined and processed foods. Simple carbohydrates include fructose (fruit sugar), sucrose (table sugar), and lactose (milk sugar). Fruit, although a simple carbohydrate, is nevertheless a vital part of eating heart-healthy provided that it's in its whole, natural state. On the other hand, fruit juices that no longer contain fiber aren't healthy for the heart. The exceptions are lemon and lime juices, which help to slow the digestion of starches (thus lowering the glycemic index of foods), and pomegranate juice, which will be discussed later.

♡ Fructose: A Weighty Issue

Overconsumption of high-sugar, high-carb foods and drinks is largely to blame for the rising rates of obesity and diabetes. But we have been so busy avoiding "sucrose" that "fructose" from corn syrup has slipped by unaware yet is also a strong contributor to these epidemics. Fructose raises blood triglycerides, VLDL cholesterol and blood sugars and contributes to liver disease, weight gain and a host of other degenerative health problems associated with carrying around those extra pounds. Read labels and avoid processed foods to reduce your fructose intake.

Complex carbohydrates include fiber and starches, which are found in vegetables, legumes, beans, nuts, seeds and whole, unrefined grains. Although you don't digest fiber, it is an important carbohydrate for lowering blood sugar, cholesterol and triglycerides.

Hearts Love Fiber
There are two types of fiber: soluble and insoluble. Soluble fiber forms a gel when mixed with liquid inside the digestive system. As it does, it locks onto cholesterol, blocking its absorption. Soluble fiber also slows the release and absorption of sugars. Insoluble fiber passes through the system largely intact. It pushes bulk through the digestive tract, preventing constipation and toxin build-up, and promoting regular elimination.

The average North American eats 10 grams or less of fiber daily. Yet dietary fiber is an excellent solution to heart and weight issues. In University of Kentucky studies, participants reduced their cholesterol by 13 to 19 percent by consuming three cups (750 mL) of cooked oat bran daily. That's a lot of oat bran! Since a diversity of foods is best, consume other fibrous sources such as oatmeal, barley, brown rice bran, fruit, vegetables, lentils and navy and pinto beans. In total, women need about 30 grams of fiber daily, and men need 35 grams. This is the equivalent found in seven to nine servings of fruit and vegetables. Various fibers are also sold as nutritional supplements. Whichever you choose, acclimate your digestive tract to increased fiber slowly to help avoid digestive distress. Also be sure to increase your water intake to aid elimination.

♡ Excellent Sources of Dietary Fiber

FOOD	SERVING SIZE	FIBER (G)
Split peas, cooked	1 cup	16.27
Lentils, cooked	1 cup	15.64
Black beans, cooked	1 cup	14.96
Green peas, boiled	1 cup	8.80
Pinto beans, cooked	1 cup	14.71
Lima beans, cooked	1 cup	13.16
Wheat, bulgur, cooked	1 cup	8.19
Kidney beans, cooked	1 cup	11.33
Barley, cooked	1 cup	13.60
Garbanzo beans (chickpeas), cooked	1 cup	12.46

The worst carbohydrates are the refined type found in cookies, cakes, crackers and desserts. Refined carbs offer empty calories and no nutrients. Your heart will thank you when you increase the number of complex carbohydrates that you eat, and reduce refined versions. If everyone stopped eating white pasta, white flour and white sugar, diabetes, high blood pressure, high cholesterol, heart disease and cancer rates would drop dramatically.

Within the complex carbohydrate category, there are foods that affect the rate of insulin release into the bloodstream. Remember, too much insulin or the fast release of insulin has health consequences and is linked to premature aging as well as to the development of diabetes and obesity, both risk factors for heart disease. To avoid this, choose mostly foods below 60 on the glycemic index. The Heart-Smart Diet isn't devoid of all carbohydrates. Instead it's based on good carbohydrates that have a lower glycemic index and don't cause rapid fluctuations in blood sugar and cause premature aging and cellular damage that invites atherosclerosis.

♡ The Low-glycemic Solution

FOOD	GLYCEMIC INDEX (GI) RATING
Glucose	100
Potato, baked	98
Carrots, cooked	92
Cornflakes	92
White rice, instant	91
Honey	74
Bread, white	72
Bagels	72
Melba toast	70
Potato, mashed	70
Bread, wheat	69
Table sugar	65
Beets	64
Raisins	61
Bran muffin	60
Pita	57

Oatmeal, large flake (not instant)	55
Popcorn (air popped)	55
Buckwheat	54
Banana	53
Brown rice	50
Grapefruit juice, unsweetened	48
Bread, whole grain pumpernickel	46
Soy milk	44
Bread, dark whole grain rye	42
Pinto beans	42
Whole grain pasta	41
Apples	39
Tomato juice, canned, unsweetened	38
All-bran cereal	38
Tomatoes	38
Yogurt, plain	38
Yams	37
Chick peas	36
Skim milk	32
Organic strawberries (i.e., pesticide-free)	32
Real egg fettuccini	32
Kidney beans	29
Whole grain spaghetti, protein-enriched	27
Peaches	26
Cherries	24
Non-starchy vegetables: arugula, asparagus, lettuces, chard, broccoli, avocado, eggplant, cucumber, cauliflower, kale, celery, all seed sprouts, Brussels sprouts, zucchini, scallions, rhubarb, purple cabbage, mushrooms	<20

Fat Phobia
Back in the 1980s, the conventional trend was to recommend a low-fat, high-carbohydrate diet for heart disease. Many of the people who followed this plan did lose weight initially, but eventually their beneficial HDL cholesterol dropped, their triglycerides flared up, and those pounds packed on again. What happened? For starters, when food companies remove fats from foods, they often replace the fats with sugar. Although a food is "non-fat" or "low-fat", it might have hundreds of calories from sugars or contain fake sugars that disrupt the body's chemistry. The sugars from a high-carb lifestyle translate into insulin resistance, which predisposes us to diabetes, premature aging, heart disease and stroke.

Plain and simple, we need fat. Fat satisfies the appetite and is essential to brain and heart function. Not all fat is created equal, however, especially when it comes to cardiovascular health. When we eat fat, the gastrointestinal tract breaks it down into triglyceride form – into free fatty acids. The fatty acids from saturated fats found in red meat and dairy products are the main source of energy production and fat storage in the body. Too much bad saturated fat, coupled with an inactive lifestyle, contributes to arterial plaque buildup and weight gain, which further stresses the heart. A diet should contain higher amounts of good fats found in healthy, cold-pressed and preferably organic oils. Good fats are liquid anti-inflammatories, soothing our arteries, eating away arterial plaque and preventing clot formation.

Not All Fats are Bad
The next time you're in the supermarket, pick up a steak and observe the fatty outer layer. What you're looking at is saturated fat, which is semisolid at room temperature and is found in animal products (red meat, pork, lamb, lard) and dairy products (milk, cheese, butter), as well as in processed foods. Saturated fats are generally considered "bad" fats that contribute to heart disease. Many health authorities

make the blanket recommendation to reduce all dietary saturated fats. However, not all saturated fats are equally deadly.

■ **The Better Saturates**

Short-chain saturates, found in butter and coconut oil, don't clog arteries, nor do they cause heart disease. Rather, they are easily digested and a source of fuel for energy. As well, short-chain saturates don't contain as many calories as longer-chain fatty acids (found in red meat).

Medium-chain saturates are found in several foods, but the highest content (just as with short-chain saturates) is found in coconut oil, and they are not associated with increasing cholesterol levels or the occurrence of heart disease.

■ **The Coconut Truth**

Coconut oil has been wrongly branded as a nutritional evil since the 1960s when research was misinterpreted and it was concluded that coconut oil raised blood cholesterol levels. In fact, it was the omission of essential fatty acids in the experimental diet that caused the observed health problems, not the inclusion of coconut oil.

Coconut oil is a short- and medium-chain fat easily digested and utilized by the body. More recent subject groups studied in the South Pacific for their regular use of dietary coconut oil exhibited low incidences of heart disease and low cholesterol levels. When our diet is rich in essential fatty acids and we consume non-hydrogenated saturate-rich coconut oil (or butter), little or no changes are evident in serum (blood) cholesterol levels. In a 2009 Brazilian study, 40 subjects involved in a randomized, double-blind, controlled clinical trial supplemented daily with 30 mL (2 Tbsp) of coconut oil; followed a balanced, calorie-reduced diet; and walked 50 minutes a day for 12 weeks. They had increases in good HDL (48.7 versus 45.0), a lower LDL-to-HDL ratio (2.41 versus 3.1) and a greater reduction in waist circumference compared to subjects who followed the same diet and fitness plan but received 30 mL (2 Tbsp) daily of soybean oil instead of coconut oil.

♡ Heart-Smart Spreads

BETTER BUTTER

1 pound (500 g) butter

1 cup (250 mL) high-quality essential fatty-acid rich oil (such as flaxseed oil, or any other organic, cold-pressed oil)

Cut butter into eight pieces. Put butter and oil into the food processor and blend until smooth. Spoon into a covered container and refrigerate. Not only will you have better butter, but it will remain soft even though refrigerated. Makes 2 cups (500 mL).

COCONUT BUTTER-FLAXSEED SPREAD

½ cup (125 mL) flaxseed oil

1 cup (250 mL) coconut butter

Place flaxseed oil in the freezer for two hours or more. Melt coconut butter on low temperature. Remove from heat. Add frozen flaxseed oil. Blend and keep in the fridge for up to six weeks. Store in an opaque container. Don't use for cooking or baking. Use as a spread in place of butter and margarine. Makes 1½ cups (375 mL).

■ *The Bad Saturates*

Long-chain saturates are the "bad" fats associated with raising LDL (the bad cholesterol), lowering HDL (the good cholesterol), and increasing the risk of heart disease. Bad saturated fats are those in red meat and dairy products. A key tenet of the Heart-Smart Diet is reducing the consumption of animal products. Long-chain saturates are also a byproduct of hydrogenation, a process that turns a liquid fat (at room temperature) into a solid and is employed in the manufacture of margarines and artificial shortenings. Long-chain saturates are also abundant in restaurant fried foods, junk food, packaged baked goods and processed foods. Hydrogenation or partial hydrogenation also distorts the fatty acids into a more toxic form for the body.

♡ Butter is Better

Butter, like eggs, has been unfairly vilified by heart disease experts. Butter contains a range of short- and medium-chain fatty acids, as well as monounsaturated and polyunsaturated fatty acids. Butter is preferable to margarine, a processed product, because butter contains many healthful components, including lecithin, which helps the body break down cholesterol. It's a rich source of vitamin A, which is necessary for healthy functioning of the adrenal and thyroid glands. The vitamins A and E and the mineral selenium in butter also serve as important antioxidants in protecting against free radical damage that can destroy tissues and weaken arterial walls. The dangers of butter's unsaturated fat components have been blown out of proportion. If used in moderation (like all good things), butter is an excellent addition to the Heart-Smart Diet, especially if improved by adding an essential fatty acid component by making Better Butter (see page 58).

The Deadliest Fats

You've likely heard of trans fatty acids, a deadly fat that task forces in the US and Canada are mandating to be removed from foods. These are formed when high temperatures and hydrogenation turn refined oils into margarines, shortenings, and partially hydrogenated vegetable oils to solidify them and give them a longer shelf life. Trans fats damage the cardiovascular system, promote cancer, impair immune function and more. Trans fats were once found in most fast foods, potato chips, French fries, baby biscuits, breakfast cereals, cookies, microwave popcorn and some margarines, to name a few. Commercially produced salad dressings can also contain trans fats as a result of the high-heat process used to make them shelf stable. Eliminate all foods that contain trans fats. Despite the efforts of food manufacturers to create trans-fat-free products, you have to read labels diligently and consider a product's fat content in context. Some potato chips may be trans-fat-free, but a potato chip is still a potato chip and is not the ideal food if you're eating for your heart and health.

Unsaturated Fats: Not Just Good but Fabulous

Unsaturated fats are liquid at room temperature and are "good" fats. They can be further classed as monounsaturated or polyunsaturated. Monounsaturated fats remain liquid at room temperature but solidify at colder temperatures. Sources of these fatty acids include olive, canola and peanut oils. Because canola is genetically modified, it is not recommended as part of the Heart-Smart Diet. Canola oil is also extensively processed, exposed to bleaching and chemical solvents that create unnatural compounds. Nor do we recommend peanut oil due to its similarly heavy refining requirements.

Extra virgin olive oil is the premium oil for the heart and should be a staple in your kitchen. The extraction method of olive oil involves careful cold-pressing to retain its beneficial properties and thousands of years of tradition. When purchasing olive oil, don't purchase those that are classified as "light;" the fair color is a good indicator that it has been processed to remove the good fats. Olive oil cannot be used in high-heat cooking. It can only be used on low heat.

Polyunsaturated fats remain liquid at room temperature, even in colder temperatures. Recommended sources of polyunsaturated fats include oils of black currant, borage, echium, flaxseed, sesame, hemp, evening primrose and fish. Unsaturated fats can be further classified as omega-3, omega-6, or omega-9. Omega-9s are monounsaturated and non-essential because we can make them from other fatty acids. Omega-3s and omega-6s are polyunsaturated and are essential because our body can't make them.

♡ Tips for Fat-tastic Eating

When shopping, choose coconut butter over lard and shortening.

Skip the margarine. Choose healthy oils that are cold-pressed and organic. Make Better Butter (see page 58).

For low-heat sautéing, use olive oil, sesame oil or coconut butter.

For salad dressings, use unrefined oils of flaxseed, hemp seed, walnut, olive, sunflower, pumpkin seed or macadamia nut.

For baking, use cold-pressed sunflower oil, butter or coconut butter.

Don't fry foods; frying promotes free radicals, which promote heart disease and other degenerative diseases. If you burn the butter in a pan or cause oil to smoke, you have created disease-promoting free radicals.

Reduce your overall consumption of animal fats.

Why We Need Essential Fats

To ward off cardiovascular disease, we must obtain beneficial essential fatty acids (EFAs) from food. They fight unhealthy cholesterol, arterial plaque and inflammation in our arteries. In the largest study examining the effect of dietary fat on heart disease risk, more than 78,000 women were followed for 20 years. Those with the highest polyunsaturated fat consumption (7.4 percent of energy), had one-quarter the heart disease risk of women with the lowest consumption (5 percent of energy).

The most abundant EFAs in the typical diet are omega-6s. Omega-6 oils are broken down into two types: Omega-6 oils that contain gamma-linolenic acid (GLA) and those that do not. Those that have GLA, including black current seed, evening primrose and borage, have been shown in clinical studies to be health protective. Those that do not contain GLA, including corn, safflower, canola and soy, have been found to be disease-promoting.

By limiting saturated fat and trans fats, and by consuming more nuts, seeds and GLA-containing omega-6 oils, you can reduce your risk of heart disease and cardiovascular-related mortality.

Omega-3 Superstars

When it comes to cardiovascular disease, the omega-3 essential fats have become nutritional superstars. These fats, which also play a role in brain function and normal growth and development, are found in fish, calamari, krill, algae, and seed oils such as flax.

Fish and fish oils started receiving mainstream support after a 1996 American Heart Association (AHA) Scientific Statement in *Circulation* noted that they reduced triglycerides in the blood and inhibited the manufacture of VLDL cholesterol, apolipoprotein B and LDL cholesterol. Omega-3s from fish were also found to reduce blood platelet stickiness; reduce blood pressure in those with hypertension or high blood cholesterol; influence blood clotting factors; reduce atherosclerotic deposits; and reduce the inflammation precursors fibrinogen and lipoprotein(a). The Nurses Health Study, which followed more than 84,000 women for 16 years, noted that women who rarely ate fish (less than once a month) had a higher risk (29 to 34 percent) of dying of coronary heart disease, and the risks dropped relative to how often the women ate fish. In another study, men who ate two fish meals a week reduced their heart attack risk by 50 percent. Other studies have noted that fish consumption protects against stroke and sudden cardiac death.

♡ Foods Concentrated in Omega-3s

FOOD	SERVING SIZE	OMEGA-3S (grams)
Flax seeds	0.25 cups	7.0 g
Walnuts	0.25 cup	2.3 g
Chinook salmon, baked/broiled	4.0 oz-wt	2.1 g
Scallops, baked/broiled	4.0 oz-wt	1.1 g
Halibut, baked/broiled	4.0 oz-wt	0.6 g
Shrimp, steamed, boiled	4.0 oz-wt	0.4 g
Snapper, baked	4.0 oz-wt	0.4 g
Winter squash	1 cup	0.3 g
Cod, baked	4.0 oz-wt	0.3 g
Kidney beans	1 cup	0.3 g

Mercury Hinders the Heart

Mercury and other heavy metals are highly toxic to the neurological system. They promote free radical formation and also hinder the body's ability to protect against free radicals. Dr. Marc Sircus, author of *Magnesium: The Ultimate Heart Medicine*, calls mercury the most potent enzyme inhibitor that exists, and how true this statement is. The heart's overall function, electrical impulse system and contractive abilities are severely impacted. Mercury is stored in the heart, where it is further implicated in oxidative stress, inflammation, endothelial and smooth muscle dysfunction, unhealthy blood fat and cholesterol levels, and more. One 2002 study of Finnish men found that those with the highest concentrations of mercury in their hair also had the highest rates of death from cardiovascular disease, heart failure and stroke.

The American Heart Association recommends eating fish twice a week but acknowledges the presence of environmental contaminants, particularly mercury, in many types of fish and seafood. The US Food and Drug Administration (FDA) advises children and women who are pregnant to avoid eating fish with the highest likely level of mercury contamination (shark, swordfish, king mackerel, tilefish); to eat up to 12 ounces (two average meals) per week of a variety of seafoods that are lower in mercury (canned light tuna, salmon, pollock, catfish). For older adults, the American Heart Association says the benefits of fish consumption outweigh the potential risks when the amount of fish eaten is within FDA recommendations. Use the calculator at www.gotmercury.org to determine a weekly suggested seafood limit based on your personal weight.

Is Your Fish Oil Green?
If you are concerned about impurities, PCBs, metals and other toxic substances in fish and fish oils but want the benefits of omega-3s, an excellent alternative is calamari oil. Calamari oil is a sustainable, eco-friendly source of omega-3 fatty acids that comes from South American calamari (squid). Calamari oil is more stable than traditional fish oils, making it less prone to rancidity. Also, calamari oil does not cause fishy burps or unpleasant "repeating" that is common with fish oil supplements. Calamari oil is much more ecologically sustainable because it comes from deep-water, spawns quickly and multiplies fast. Because of their short life span, calamari does not have the same issues with mercury and heavy metal toxicity that fish do. Furthermore, calamari oil is a better alternative to fish oil because it contains much more DHA.

Docosahexaenoic acid (DHA)
DHA (docosahexaenoic acid) is an important omega-3 fatty acid essential for the brain, nervous system, eyes and heart. Many vegetarians, vegans and raw food dieters are deficient in DHA unless they supplement with vegetarian algae DHA. Mother's milk contains high amounts of DHA to ensure proper brain development in an infant. Calamari oil contains both EPA and DHA but it is the fact that it has a high amount of DHA that makes it an omega-3 superstar.

DHA for High Triglycerides

A 2009 double-blind study published in the *Journal of Nutrition* showed that men with elevated triglycerides had lower levels of C-reactive protein (CRP), a marker for inflammation, after taking DHA every day compared to those taking a placebo. We know that high triglycerides are linked to hardening of the arteries and an increased risk of dying from cardiovascular disease. Elevated CRP is a risk factor for heart attack (see page 32 for more on CRP). By taking DHA, CRP was lowered by over 15 percent.

Another study performed at the Western Human Nutrition Research Center found that DHA supplementation over 4 months decreased triglycerides by about 26 percent and increased good HDL cholesterol by approximately 9 percent. The researchers also looked at indicators for bleeding and blood clotting. Fish oils have been shown to increase bleeding times and inhibit clotting but high doses of DHA did not, thus making a higher dose of DHA a safer option.

According to a meta-analysis of randomized, placebo-controlled trials that compared DHA to EPA, researchers found that DHA was superior at reducing elevated triglycerides. This is another reason to use calamari oil which is high in DHA.

DHA and High Blood Pressure

A study in 1999 in *Hypertension* showed that DHA but not EPA lowered high blood pressure.

DHA and High Cholesterol

A study published in *Lipids* evaluated the effects of DHA-rich fish oils in 45 patients with high cholesterol treated with statin medications. Patients were randomized to three groups and they were either given 4 g/day or 8 g/day of tuna oil containing DHA or a placebo for 6 months. DHA supplementation as an adjunct to statin therapy produced a greater cholesterol reduction in the patients than statin use alone.

DHA and Memory

DHA makes up 40 percent of the essential fats in your brain. DHA supplementation supports the central nervous system and enhances cognition. Now researchers are investigating the benefits of DHA in patients with Alzheimer's and dementia. Observational data published in the *American Journal of Clinical Nutrition* suggests that consuming at least 180 mg of DHA on a daily basis could reduce the risk of dementia by almost 50 percent. Make Cala-Q Plus your DHA supplement providing 720 mg of DHA per serving. Additional observational data from the massive Framingham Heart Study showed that high DHA can improve mental function, reduce cognitive decline, and stave off Alzheimer's.

DHA and Your Vision

DHA is the best fatty acid for eye health and dry eyes. Over 30 percent of the retina is made up of DHA. The *British Journal of Opthamology* found that DHA helped to prevent macular degeneration, the leading cause of blindness today. I can't think of anyone who is not concerned about their vision. DHA fatty acid rich oils also help to moisturize dry eyes as well.

♡ **Healthy Fats and Oils**

Brazil nuts	Pine nuts
Pumpkin seeds	Sunflower seeds
Sesame seeds	Black current seed
Evening primrose	Borage
Echium	Flax
Fish	Olive oil
Hemp seed	Calamari

IN MODERATION:

Butter	Coconut oil

Sound Cardiology Advice

If you're an Oprah fan, perhaps you caught the episode where TV personality and cardiologist Dr. Mehmet Oz discussed the revelatory results of a study looking at diet and heart disease risk factors. Eating 11 pounds of fruits, vegetables and nuts a day is no small amount. However, after 12 days, this nutritional abundance dropped participants' cholesterol by an average of 25 percent, their blood pressure dropped by 10 percent, and they lost 10 pounds each, including more than two inches around their waists. Dr. Oz says most white foods should be avoided because they're made of predominantly processed, simple carbohydrates that spike blood sugar levels and stress the cardiovascular system. To support the heart, Dr. Oz also prescribes a high-protein breakfast that will curb carbohydrate cravings. He also suggests eating a small portion of protein 20 minutes before big meals to prevent overeating and mid-meal cravings.

Quality protein is an important part of the Heart-Smart Diet. Faced with a pork hot dog and a skinless chicken breast, which would you imagine is healthier? Naturally, the latter is better because it's leaner, lower in saturated fats, unprocessed, and (ideally) free range or organic. Combined with low-glycemic carbohydrates and good fats, protein from lean meats, eggs, poultry, fish, seafood and protein powders provide the body with amino acid fuel.

Our body requires 20 essential amino acids in the production of protein for cellular repair, the manufacture of hormones, immune system factors, enzymes and tissues. Of those 20 amino acids, 12 can be made within the body and the remaining eight must be obtained from food. Two groups of proteins are found in the diet. Complete proteins – including meat, fish, poultry, cheese, eggs, milk, fermented soy and whey protein powders – contain all the essential amino acids. Incomplete proteins – including grains, legumes, and leafy green vegetables – don't contain all the essential amino acids.

The Protein Difference

A 2006 study in the *New England Journal of Medicine* confirmed that women who follow a diet lower in carbohydrates and higher in vegetable fat and protein have a reduced risk of heart disease. More than 82,000 women in the Nurses Health Study filled out dietary questionnaires and were followed for 20 years. Researchers noted that women with the lowest carb intake and the highest intake of vegetable proteins and fats had a 30 percent lower risk of coronary heart disease compared to women who ate the most carbs and fewest proteins and fats from vegetable sources. They also found that a higher glycemic (sugar) load in the body also increased the risk of heart disease.

A more recent study confirmed the importance of proper protein choices. After analyzing data collected between 1995 and 2005 involving more than 500,000 men and women between the ages of 50 and 71, US researchers at the National Cancer Institute found that people whose diets are high in processed and red meats are more likely to die from cancer or heart disease. Those who ate 8.5 4-ounce servings of red meat weekly (beef, hamburger, cold cuts, liver, sausage, pork, prepared meats in items like lasagne and pizza) had a 30 percent higher mortality rate than those who ate one weekly serving of meat. In heavy meat-eating men, cancer and cardiovascular-related deaths increased 22 and 27 percent respectively. In women who were heavy meat eaters, the death rates increased by 20 percent for cancer and 50 percent for heart disease. The study, published in 2009 in the *Archives of Internal Medicine*, is much broader in scope than previous studies comparing death rates of meat eaters.

♡ **Make Protein a Top Pick**

- Eat more cold-water fish or seafood than red meat.
- Choose wild fish over farmed fish.

- Choose organic and free-range poultry and eggs over conventionally raised.
- Eat vegetarian proteins including legumes such as beans, chickpeas and lentils.
- Purchase raw (unroasted), unsalted nuts and seeds.
- Remove all visible fat from meat prior to cooking.
- Choose extra-lean ground chicken, turkey and beef. Choose leaner cuts of steak, e.g. sirloin, tenderloin, top round.
- Broiling, baking, steaming and grilling are better than frying and deep-frying.
- Reduce your dairy intake.

The Heart-Smart plate should be abundant in nutrient-rich greenery with EFA-rich oils and salad dressings. It should be low in processed, high-glycemic carbohydrates, and should be finished off with a piece of quality protein about the size of your palm. Some people do have greater protein needs than others. If you're very active, exercise strenuously or do heavy labor, or if you're pregnant, you'll need more protein than if you're a couch potato. And since our goal is to get you up and active, be sure not to neglect your protein needs!

How Much Protein Do You Need?

Adult men	70 g
Adult women	58 g
Pregnant women	65 g
Lactating women	75 g
Girls aged 13-15	62 g
Girls aged 16-20	58 g
Boys aged 13-15	75 g
Boys aged 16-20	85 g

The Soy Story
Soybeans, soy milk, tofu, miso and tempeh are rich protein sources
known for their cholesterol-lowering properties. Soy foods, 25 grams
daily, can also lower triglycerides, raise HDL cholesterol, inhibit
cholesterol oxidation and inhibit blood clotting. The US Food and
Drug Administration allows soy foods with 6.25 grams or more per
serving to carry a heart-health claim on their label. However, not
all soy is the same.

Fermented soy includes miso, tempeh, soy sauce, and fermented
soy powders. Traditional Asian diets contain mainly fermented
soy foods, not isolated soy protein, soy milk or whole soybeans.
Non-fermented soy foods block the production of protein-derived
hormones, inhibit thyroid hormone uptake and contain phytic
acid, which can inhibit nutrient absorption. Most non-fermented
soy products are also genetically modified, unless the label clearly
states otherwise. In contrast, the fermentation process deacti-
vates many of soy's detrimental effects. Fermented soy isoflavones
aren't as strong as conventional isoflavones, which may stimulate
estrogen-receptor cells in breast tissue. However, controversy
over soy's effect on abnormal cell growth lingers. For this reason,
fermented soy foods only in moderation are recommended and
women with estrogen-receptor-positive breast cancer should
avoid all soy products. There exist plenty of other quality sources
to satisfy your protein needs.

Eat Like a Mediterranean
Ah, the Mediterranean – famous for its pristine beaches, magnif-
icent scenery, holiday magic and, last but not least, its delicious
food. Over the past several years, researchers have focused more
and more of their attention on how the components of traditional
Mediterranean cuisine put it at the head of the pack at disease-
prevention and preserving longevity. Not surprisingly given the fact
that Mediterranean populations enjoy one of the lowest rates of

heart disease in the world, their diet is based on fresh, unprocessed foods that support heart health:

- Abundant fruits and vegetables, which are rich in vitamins and minerals (e.g. vitamins C and E, magnesium, zinc, l-gluta-thione) as well as powerful plant elements (phytochemicals) known to fight cancer, and heart and eye disease;
- Low-glycemic legumes (lentils, chickpeas) that metabolize into sugar slowly and don't require the pancreas to produce as much insulin, thus protecting against the irregular sugar metabolism associated with (pre)diabetic states, high cholesterol and hypertension;
- Rich in root vegetables (garlic, onions) whose antioxidant properties fight free radical damage, and help to lower blood pressure;
- Higher consumption of seafood and fish, which contain essential fatty acids that support cardiovascular health;
- Healthy fat choices, with olive oil being the primary food oil;
- Traditional food preparation that retains food's nutritive properties; e.g. foods picked riper, which allow higher nutrient development, and less frying and deep frying, which cuts down on dangerous trans fat consumption;
- Lowered meat and dairy intake, i.e. less artery-damaging saturated fat and methionine, the precursor to homocysteine, high levels of which is an undesirable marker for heart disease;
- More fiber-rich whole grains, fruits and vegetables that help stabilize blood sugar and support digestive health;
- Fewer processed, high-glycemic carbohydrates (e.g. white bread, white pasta) that throw off blood sugar, contribute to weight gain, encourage insulin resistance and create fatty, sticky blood;
- Red wine, which contains arterial-plaque-preventive quercetin and the phytochemical resveratrol, which has captured media spotlight for its antioxidant capacities.

Preserve Heart Longevity

In study after study, the traditional Mediterranean diet has justified its celebrity health status. It prevents heart disease and reduces the risk of future cardiac events such as heart attacks and cardiac death due to its positive effect on various risk factors, including high blood pressure, diabetes, obesity and high cholesterol. The Mediterranean diet also lowers LDL oxidation and cellular fat levels.

Researchers looking at more than 9,400 Spanish men and women reported earlier this year that a Mediterranean-type diet was also associated with reduced systolic and diastolic blood pressure. They assessed diet using questionnaires and a six-year follow-up and concluded that "adhering to a Mediterranean-type diet could contribute to the prevention of age-related changes in blood pressure." Eating like a Mediterranean also improves blood sugar regulation, helps reduce the prevalence of metabolic syndrome and reduces inflammatory markers.

Powerful Pomegranate

Pomegranate packs a powerful nutritional punch. The fruit is a many-seeded berry and is surrounded by a juicy, fleshy outer layer. The seeds possess anti-inflammatory properties by inhibiting enzymes responsible for inflammation and pain. Pomegranate juice has antioxidant power close to that of green tea and significantly greater than red wine. The juice has been shown to offer protection against cardiovascular disease by reducing:
- cholesterol accumulation
- the development of atherosclerosis
- systolic blood pressure
- stress-induced myocardial ischemia in patients who have coronary heart disease
- thickening of the carotid artery.

A 2004 study in *Clinical Nutrition* found that 19 patients with severe atherosclerosis of the carotid arteries who drank two ounces of pomegranate juice daily for three years had remarkable results. Ultrasound tests showed that narrowing of the arteries decreased by 35 percent on average in the pomegranate group, while the condition worsened by nearly 10 percent in the control group. The average systolic blood pressure was also significantly lowered in the group who drank pomegranate juice.

Pomegranate juice extract improves clinical gum disease, a precursor and/or indication of cardiovascular disease. In another study, it reduced the harmful products of lipid (fat) oxidation in the blood in diabetic patients without affecting insulin levels. Israeli researchers also reported in the journal *Atherosclerosis* that 50 mL of juice daily for three months slowed oxidative stress and the development of atherosclerosis in type 2 diabetics. Although pomegranate juice contains sugars, it didn't affect the patients' serum glucose levels.

♡ Heart Superfoods

Flaxseeds	Berries
Pumpkin seeds	Apples
Olives	Spinach
Walnuts	Shitake
Almonds	Beans and lentils
Quinoa	Salmon
Pomegranate	Prunes

Dangerously Sugary Drinks

Regular consumption of sugary beverages increases heart disease risk. In a recent *American Journal of Clinical Nutrition* study involving 89,000 healthy women between 34 and 59 years old, one sugar-sweetened drink daily increased the risk of heart disease by 23 percent, and two or more drinks daily increased it by 35 percent compared with women who consumed less than one sweetened drink per month.

Habitual consumption of high-sugar beverages and foods contributes to irregular sugar metabolism, insulin resistance, diabetes and metabolic syndrome, which are all linked to heart disease. Too much sugar lowers protective HDL and raises blood pressure. Sugar orders the liver to produce triglycerides; the more you eat, the more triglyceride levels rise. Sugary foods represent extra calories that we must work harder to burn off.

Red, Red Wine

Alcohol is a common source of dietary sugar. True, antioxidant-rich red wine is widely touted for heart health. Moderate consumption is thought to reduce heart disease by increasing good HDL cholesterol and by reducing blood platelet clumping and clotting. However, two or more drinks a day raise blood pressure, and given alcohol's other health effects (e.g. boosting blood sugar, disabling detoxification), only an occasional drink is part of the Heart-Smart Diet. If you want the benefits of resveratrol, choose another source such as red grapes, blueberries, cranberries or resveratrol in supplement form.

Breakfast Bevvies

When it comes to coffee, that cup o' Joe might boost energy, improve endurance and prompt alertness, but too much can also cause headaches, indigestion and tremors, and is linked to osteoporosis, infertility and incontinence. Caffeine from coffee and other sources (soft drinks, medications) stimulates the nervous system and can affect heart rate. Five or more cups a day is associated with a 2.4/1.2 mmHg increase in blood pressure. Coffee can also raise levels of homocysteine, which damages arteries and promotes atherosclerosis and blood clots.

Tea, on the other hand, contains many heart-friendly compounds – flavonoids, tannins, catechins. In women, daily tea consumption has been found to reduce carotid plaque. A review of studies between

between 1990 and 2004 confirmed that three cups of black tea daily reduced the risk of heart disease. Regular tea drinkers have a lower risk of heart attack; the same effect isn't seen with regular and decaffeinated coffee. Green and white teas lead the tea troupe because they have more antioxidants and catechins than black tea. Research on the fat-fighting, blood lipid-lowering and anti-cancer effects of these powerful teas continues.

Herbal hibiscus tea has hearty benefits. Three cups of hibiscus tea daily for six weeks reduces systolic blood pressure, according to research from Tufts University presented at the American Heart Association Scientific Sessions in November 2008. Among those patients with a systolic reading over the median of 129 mmHg, hibiscus tea consumption reduced it by 14 mmHg. Participants at or below 129 mmHg had an average drop of 7 mmHg. On a population basis, a 3 mmHg reduction would yield an 8 percent drop in stroke mortality and a 5 percent drop in heart disease mortality, highlighting the importance that this one tea could make.

The Sodium-Potassium Connection
There is much focus on the connection between sodium (salt) and elevated blood pressure. Abundant effort has also been put on salt reduction as part of blood pressure management. For instance, one landmark study, the DASH-Sodium Trial, assigned over 400 people with prehypertension and hypertension (prehypertension = 130–139/85–89 mmHg, hypertension = >140/>90) to either the standard American diet or the DASH diet. In the DASH diet group, blood pressure dropped nicely and this was largely attributed to a reduced sodium intake. However, salt is not the real culprit when it comes to high blood pressure. The true issue is that we are not consuming enough potassium and magnesium along with sodium. While the DASH diet does reduce sodium, it also contains more vegetables that provide minerals in which many people are deficient. Instead of doctors recommending to their patients to reduce salt

consumption, their focus should be on encouraging patients to increase the amount of potassium and magnesium in the diet.

We need sodium to modulate muscle and nerve function, and to regulate our fluid balance and blood pressure. In northern countries like Canada and in the northern United States, the main source of iodine in the diet is from iodized salts. So when we tell people to avoid all salt, we get a corresponding rise in cases of low thyroid function because the thyroid needs iodine (the reason iodine was added to salt was to improve the function of the thyroid). The key to optimal heart health is that we just don't need more salt than potassium and magnesium. Most North Americans ingest twice as much sodium compared to potassium. Some Americans consume up to 20 grams of sodium a day! But the body needs five times as much potassium as sodium. Potassium supplements would not be necessary if we simply ate more vegetables (seven to 10 half-cup servings to be exact). Most vegetables contain 50 times more potassium than sodium. As an example, the ratio of potassium-to-sodium is:

• Apples, 90:1
• Bananas, 440:1
• Carrots, 75:1
• Oranges, 260:1
• Potatoes, 110:1.

Multipurpose Heart Mineral
Magnesium is beneficial in improving heart rates in heart failure patients and in improving survival rates and clinical symptoms and quality of life in heart patients with severe congestive heart failure. It reduces C-reactive protein levels (a marker of inflammation) and improves exercise tolerance, exercise-induced chest pain and quality of life in patients with coronary artery disease, and much more. Its relaxing effect makes magnesium valuable in cases of arrhythmia – even in life-threatening situations, research has shown. One study looking at magnesium treatment immediately

after heart attack found that it slashed the death rate by 75 percent and resulted in fewer complications in 96 patients. A 2005 meta-analysis of randomized, controlled trials involving magnesium use on patients with an irregular heartbeat (atrial fibrillation) after heart surgery, found that fewer patients in the magnesium groups developed post-operative irregular heartbeats compared to the control groups (18 versus 28 percent).

Magnesium-rich foods include whole grains, legumes and vegetables. Older adults are more at risk because magnesium absorption is affected by age. Dietary surveys reveal that most North Americans don't even get the RDA of magnesium, which hovers between 300 and 400 mg for teenagers and adults. RDAs are not sufficient for optimal health; we need much more than the RDA.

♡ Recommended Foods with Magnesium

FOOD	SERVING SIZE	AMOUNT (MG)
Swiss chard, boiled	1 cup	151
Spinach, boiled	1 cup	157
Pumpkin seeds, raw	0.25 cup	185
Halibut, baked/broiled	4 oz-wt	121
Sunflower seeds, raw	0.25 cup	127
Sesame seeds	0.25 cup	126
Black beans, cooked	1 cup	120
Salmon, chinook, baked/broiled	4 oz-wt	138
Navy beans, cooked	1 cup	107
Millet, cooked	1 cup	106

Eat with Mindfulness

Food is a miracle, life-sustaining and the connection between the natural world and ourselves. Let's treat our food and bodies respectfully.

Eat in a calm, quiet atmosphere. Turn off the TV and phone, keeping your focus on your meal.

Chew food thoroughly. Racing through a meal without proper chewing forces our digestive organs to work harder.

Eat freshly cooked meals. Aim for balance, with fruits and vegetables as ripe as possible for maximum nutrient content.

Stop when you're almost full. By setting down your fork when you're 75 percent full, you avoid overeating and stressing your digestive system.

Make the time to enjoy food. Even if it's only 20 minutes, appreciate quality mealtime, including a few minutes afterward of relaxation to aid digestion.

chapter eight

Heart-Smart Nutrients

Many nutritionists and dietitians advise us that we can get adequate nutritional requirements from the foods we eat. "Adequate" nutrition is just not good enough anymore – especially if we want to prevent or treat heart disease. People often resist making diet changes or adding nutrients until a health crisis forces them to rethink what their body needs. In a perfect world, you could obtain all the nutrients you need from the foods you eat, but today most people are eating the "SAD" – the Standard American Diet. For example, how many people eat the seven to 10 half-cup (875-1,250 mL) servings of vegetables and fruits needed just to get the minimum basic nutrients for adequate health? Over 80 percent of North Americans eat two servings of vegetables per day – one of these being French fries. With our exposure to environmental pollutants, stress, aging and illness, we need even more vitamins, minerals, fatty acids and coenzymes to keep disease at bay. You are most likely reading this book because you already have some heart disease risks.

Cardiovascular nutrient research is an exciting area of study with excellent clinical human research to show how effective nutrients are at not only preventing heart disease but also treating existing cardiovascular problems. There are dozens of nutrients on the market for heart disease. The following key nutrients have been chosen for their scientific validity, safety and effectiveness.

Sytrinol Lowers Cholesterol and Triglycerides in 30 Days
Sytrinol is a safe, effective cholesterol- and triglyceride-lowering nutrient that works in 30 days. It's comprised of a patented blend of powerful antioxidants including polymethoxylated flavones (PMFs) and a range of palm (alpha, delta and gamma) tocotrienols. Studies have revealed that sytrinol is able to significantly lower total cholesterol, bad cholesterol (LDL) and triglycerides. Better still, this proprietary ingredient has also been shown to increase good cholesterol (HDL) levels.

Sytrinol Keeps Arteries Clear
Polymethoxylated flavones (PMFs), one of the main active ingredients in sytrinol, are a group of compounds derived from the peels of citrus fruits. The two most common are tangeretin and nobiletin, which are extremely potent bioflavonoids. More than 25 years of documented research provides evidence that these particular bioflavonoids deliver heart health benefits.

Nobiletin and tangeretin help lower levels of bad LDL by blocking the enzymes in the liver responsible for the manufacture of its building blocks: apolipoprotein B and triglycerides. Apolipoprotein B is considered the primary building block of bad cholesterol, making up almost 90 per cent of LDL cholesterol. Interestingly, triglycerides, the main kind of fat in your body, are one of the key contributors to the formation of apolipoprotein B.

Sytrinol is also comprised of palm tocotrienols, which, like tocopherols, are members of the vitamin E family and are extracted from the fruit of the palm tree. The palm tocotrienols in sytrinol come from Malaysia, a world leader in palm fruit sustainable farming. Like vitamin E, palm tocotrienols control anti-inflammatory responses and degrade HMG-CoA reductase, a key enzyme in your body used by your liver to produce cholesterol. Besides reducing cholesterol, palm tocotrienols have also been shown to inhibit arterial plaque formation and reduce your blood from clumping (platelet aggregation).

Sytrinol Is a Powerful Antioxidant

Palm tocotrienols are also powerful antioxidants, known to possess antioxidant potential far greater than that shown by vitamin E itself. In human studies, it was observed that alpha tocotrienols decreased the oxidation of bad LDL. This action is important as high levels of LDL is a risk factor in cardiovascular disease. The antioxidant properties of tocotrienols can minimize the damage caused by these compounds while protecting cell membranes.

Clinical results have shown that sytrinol exerts effects very similar to cholesterol-lowering statin drugs but without side-effects.

Sytrinol Improves LDL:HDL Ratio

To date, three main studies have been carried out to investigate sytrinol's effects on high cholesterol levels. The first study involved 60 participants with raised cholesterol levels. After taking 300 mg of sytrinol each day for four weeks, the researchers found that sytrinol lowered total cholesterol by 25 percent, the bad LDL cholesterol by 19 percent, and triglycerides by 24 percent.

In the second, smaller study 10 subjects with elevated cholesterol levels benefited after four weeks of treatment with 300 mg of sytrinol per day. Sytrinol therapy lowered total cholesterol levels by 20 percent, LDL cholesterol by 22 percent, apolipoprotein B (a component of LDL) by 21 percent, and triglycerides by 28 percent. Participants also had a significant five percent increase in apolipoprotein A1, an important structural protein of the good HDL cholesterol.

Researchers have now completed a third clinical trial, a 12-week placebo-controlled study involving 120 men and women with moderately elevated cholesterol levels. Compared to those in the placebo group, subjects taking sytrinol had a 30 percent drop in total cholesterol, a 27 percent drop in LDL cholesterol, and a 34 percent drop in triglycerides. In addition, HDL levels increased by 4 percent, resulting in a significant 29 percent improvement in the LDL:HDL ratio.

The best news is that sytrinol worked independently of diet changes. Toxicity studies have shown that sytrinol is well tolerated, with no toxic effects following consumption of up to one percent of total dietary intake, or the equivalent of a 150-pound person consuming almost 14 grams per day – that's nearly 50 times the recommended daily dosage of sytrinol at 300 mg per day.

Four human clinical trials have demonstrated that sytrinol reduced total cholesterol by 30 percent, LDL cholesterol by 27 percent, and triglycerides by 34 percent when compared to placebo in 30 days.

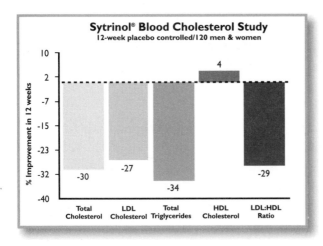

Sytrinol's Five Actions Maintain a Healthy Heart
■ *Total Cholesterol Benefits*
Sytrinol's tocotrienols work by inhibiting the rate-limiting enzyme HMG-CoA reductase in the liver. However, sytrinol's mode of

action contrasts with the competitive inhibition of HMG-CoA reductase receptors exhibited by statin drugs. The cholesterol-lowering effect of sytrinol appears to act by a novel process that controls the degradation rate of the HMG-CoA reductase enzyme. In other words, rather than actually preventing the manufacture of HMG-CoA reductase enzyme, which statin drugs do, the tocotrienols in sytrinol reduce the levels of this important enzyme required for cholesterol by increasing the rate at which the enzyme molecules degrade. As a result, sytrinol increases the rate of natural degradation of HMG-CoA reductase and reduces total cholesterol without the side-effects associated with statins.

Cardiovascular Prescription Drugs

COMMON SIDE-EFFECTS	
Cholesterol Lowering Drugs	**High Blood Pressure Drugs**
Muscle pain	Depression
Destruction of CoQ10	Kidney damage
Liver damage	Palpitations
Abdominal pain	Rapid heart rate
Constipation pain	Constipation
Gas	Insomnia
Kidney damage	Impotence

■ LDL Benefits

Sytrinol's PMFs are known to reduce both apolipoprotein B levels needed for the manufacture of LDL particles and reduce levels of microsomal triglyceride transfer protein, which is needed to transfer fat into the bad LDL particles.

■ Triglyceride Benefits

PMFs are known to reduce DGAT activity (diacylglycerol acetyltransferase) and increase liver PPAR (peroxisome proliferator activated receptor) – and in doing so, reduce the overall manufacture of triglycerides (DGAT inhibition) and increase fatty acid oxidation, thereby reducing triglyceride levels in the blood by two complementary mechanisms.

■ *Anti-inflammatory Benefits*

Inflammation, as we have learned, is a major trigger in heart disease. Studies are showing that heart disease is afflicting younger and younger people. One third of those are in good health and their cholesterol is within normal ranges. Both men and women in this group have been shown to suffer from sudden heart attacks with no warning signs or risk factors known to cause heart disease. As you read earlier, recent research has established that inflammation may be the cause, as inflammation causes C-reactive protein (CRP), which is a known marker for sudden heart attack, to be produced in the body. Researchers have shown that the presence of CRP in the body is a more reliable predictor of a pending heart attack than any other traditionally known risk factor for heart disease.

The PMFs nobiletin and tangeretin have been studied for their anti-inflammatory properties, showing that the PMFs found in sytrinol would have a positive effect on CRP.

■ *Antioxidant Benefits*

PMFs and tocotrienols are among many natural potent antioxidants that have been researched for decades. PMFs can help protect blood vessel linings and prevent the oxidation of bad LDL cholesterol, which can lead to cardiovascular disease. Tocotrienols reduce oxidative damage, as well as reduce the incidence of chronic diseases such as heart disease and cancer.

♡ Statins Expensive and Dangerous

Statins are the number one selling prescription drug in the North America today. Statins are typically used to lower cholesterol and belong to a drug category known as HMG-CoA reductase inhibitors. Commonly used branded drugs in this category include: atorvastatin (Lipitor), cerivastatin (Baycol), lovastatin (Mevacor), pravastatin (Pravachol), rosuvastatin (Crestor) and simvastatin (Zocor). They are also costly, and depending on dosage, (the dosage range is 10-80 mg per day), their use is estimated at $3-8 per day or $90-240 per month. Statins are typically prescribed with the goal of lowering LDL cholesterol. They work on inhibiting cholesterol manufacture and increasing the number of LDL receptors in the liver. Use of statins is not without risk, however; some side-effects are:

- Muscle pain, weakness and damage
- Nerve damage
- Measurable decline in cognition
- Increased risk of cancer
- Liver problems
- Joint pain
- Heart failure
- Muscle inflammation
- Stains are disruptive to the natural overall balance of the body, blocking the natural production of coenzyme Q10 which share the same metabolic pathway affected by statins.

Sytrinol is not only advantageous compared to statin medications, but it has also been shown to be a superior therapy in its ability to safely reduce cholesterol without dangerous side effects. Even some natural remedies have potential problems. For example, red yeast rice, a common cholesterol-lowering natural remedy, is almost identical to prescription statins in chemical structure and blocks the same pathway. Adding to consumer safety concerns, Consumer Labs reported that 40 percent of red yeast rice products tested in the US contained toxic citrinin, and the amount of lovastatin (statin drug) in each product varied more than 100-fold. A UCLA study supports the Consumer Labs' findings as it showed that only one of nine red yeast rice supplements bought in health food stores contained all the monacolins that lower cholesterol, and seven of nine red yeast rice supplements contained measurable concentrations of toxic citrinin. Canada has banned red yeast rice extracts. In the US, the FDA has taken the position that "red yeast rice products containing standardized lovastatin levels are unapproved new drugs." Clearly, red yeast rice has been, and continues to be, under heavy regulatory scrutiny and safety concerns persist.

Sytrinol daily dose: 300 mg per day with or without food.

Sytrinol should not be taken with sterols, another natural remedy for improving your lipid profile (triglycerides and cholesterol), because sterols inhibit their absorption and reduce their effectiveness.

Pine Bark Extract Protects the Heart
Standardized extract from the bark of the French maritime pine tree (*Pinus pinaster*) contains a potent blend of active phenolic compounds including catechins, taxifolium, procyanidins and phenolic acids. French maritime pine bark extract is known to be one of the most potent antioxidant compounds currently known. In fact, research has demonstrated that pine bark extract is up to 100 times more powerful than vitamin E. Pine bark extract is extremely effective at inactivating and neutralizing free radicals (molecules that damage any structure they come into contact with). And pine bark extract has the ability to recycle and prolong the life span of key antioxidant vitamins C and E. Antioxidants protect against the cell-damaging effects of free radicals. Free radicals, as we learned earlier, are by-products of normal physiological processes like digestion, for example, and their production can

be exacerbated by lifestyle and environmental factors. Since free radicals are considered a major cause of aging and play a key role in the development of age-related diseases such as heart disease and dementia, the use of powerful antioxidants like pine bark extract may counteract some of the problems associated with aging.

French maritime pine bark extract helps:
- prevent blood clots
- protect DNA from damage
- lower blood sugar levels when elevated
- normalize high blood pressure
- reduce the risk of cancer
- protect cells from the damage of UV radiation
- protect against the damaging effects of cigarette smoke
- improve sperm quality
- improve wound healing
- improve lung function in asthmatics
- ease menstrual cramps.

Pine Bark Extract Lowers High Blood Pressure
Research examining the effects of pine bark extract on high blood pressure showed it significantly lowered blood pressure in patients with moderately high blood pressure. Two hundred milligrams of French maritime pine bark extract daily was enough to have a dramatic reduction on both systolic and diastolic blood pressure. It is believed that pine bark's ability to elevate nitric oxide production is the primary reason for reduced blood pressure. Nitric oxide causes blood vessels to relax, increasing blood flow and decreasing blood pressure. Pine bark extract has also been researched in people with moderately high blood pressure as well.

Pine Bark Extract – Blood Clot Preventer
French maritime pine bark is also effective at reducing blood clots. Belcaro and researchers evaluated the risk of deep vein thrombosis

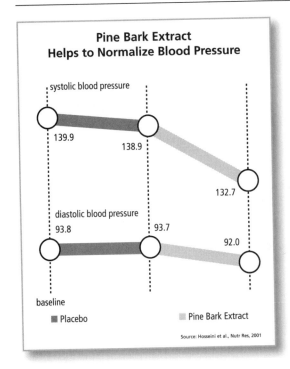

**Pine Bark Extract
Helps to Normalize Blood Pressure**

systolic blood pressure

139.9

138.9

132.7

diastolic blood pressure

93.8   93.7

92.0

baseline

■ Placebo   ▨ Pine Bark Extract

Source: Hosseini et al., Nutr Res, 2001

**Double-blind, placebo-
controlled cross-over
study with borderline
hypertensive patients
not taking hypertensive
medication.**

(DVT) during flights longer than eight hours. Those participants using French maritime pine bark extract had no cases of deep vein thrombosis whereas, in the group taking a placebo, there were five cases of thrombosis. Like previous research, it is believed that pine bark's ability to relax blood vessels (which increases blood flow) is the reason for reduced blood clots. Other research has also shown that French maritime pine bark extract reduces the stickiness of the blood. Reducing the risk of blood clots is particularly important since we know blood clots can cause strokes and heart attacks. Every 35 seconds in North America someone has a stroke.

Pine Bark Extract Repairs Capillaries

As we age, our blood vessels loose their elasticity and can leak. French maritime pine bark repairs damaged blood vessels by enhancing collagen. Collagen is the component that makes our skin smooth, nails, hair and bones strong, and it also provides shape and flexibility to our blood vessels, capillaries and veins – all part of a healthy cardiovascular system.

Pine Bark Extract Prevents Fat Deposition in Artery Walls

Fatty deposits in our arteries are a major factor in coronary artery disease. French maritime pine bark extract can also help to prevent the buildup of fatty deposits in artery walls. When LDL, the bad cholesterol, is oxidized, it becomes sticky and accumulates on the inner lining of blood vessels. Blood flow is reduced as the deposits become thicker. When this occurs to the capillaries supplying the heart, it can lead to a heart attack if blood supply is completely blocked. French maritime pine bark was found to reduce the oxidation of LDL cholesterol and prevent the buildup of fatty deposits.

Pine bark extract daily dose: 30-200 mg per day with meals.

For those persons with both high cholesterol and high blood pressure, a combination of sytrinol and pine bark effectively lowers both conditions.

Coenzyme Q10 – The Heart Superstar

Coenzyme Q10 or ubiquinone, often referred to as CoQ10 or Q10, is one of the most powerful antioxidants known for helping maintain a healthy heart. Although CoQ10 has been described as a coenzyme, it functions more like a vitamin. Vitamins by definition are essential and coenzyme CoQ10 is a micronutrient that supports biochemical reactions in the body. Coenzyme Q10 is produced naturally by the body, but production declines as we age. By 50, everyone should be taking a daily supplement of CoQ10.

Coenzyme Q10 exists in the mitochondria, the powerhouse of our cells. CoQ10 enhances energy at the cellular level, especially in the heart, enabling your heart muscle to pump blood efficiently. With the help of CoQ10, ATP (adenosine triphosphate) is made inside the mitochondria and provides the fuel that gives the entire body energy. CoQ10 acts as the battery charger for the energy system in the heart and other body cells. The heart is one of the few organs that never takes a rest, continuously functioning. This is the main reason CoQ10 is probably the single best nutrient that you can take for a healthy heart.

Statin Drugs Deplete CoQ10

Statin drugs inhibit the body's manufacture of CoQ10 just like they do cholesterol, so the reduction of CoQ10 in the body when taking statins is not a side-effect but an inherent function of the statin drugs. Statin drugs can decrease the body's manufacture of CoQ10 by as much as 40 percent. It is imperative if you are taking statin drugs that you supplement with CoQ10 daily. In May 2007, the *American Journal of Cardiology* reported a study of 32 patients with muscle symptoms associated with the use of statins. The patients were randomly divided into two groups. For one month, one group took daily CoQ10 at a dosage of 100 mg while the other took 400 IU (international units) of vitamin E daily. After 30 days, the patients who received CoQ10 experienced a 40 percent reduction in the severity of pain associated with statin use. No significant changes were found among those who received vitamin E.

Statins Increase Breast Cancer Risk

Statin medication use is also associated with breast cancer. One study in the *Procedures of the American Society of Clinical Oncology* found that the incidence of breast cancer increases when women use statin medications. A total of 66,843 women over the age of 35 were included in the study. Statin use was identified from pharmacy data collected from 1997 until 2002. Statins were found to increase estrogen levels in women. The average age of women in the research group taking statins who developed breast cancer was 58 years. The researchers reported that women taking statin medications should be advised of the potential increased risk of breast cancer.

> ## Multipurpose CoQ10
>
> Not only does CoQ10 provide a strong, healthy heart, but it also helps:
> - Maintain a healthy cholesterol ratio
> - Protect all cellular membranes
> - Halt free radical damage due to its powerful antioxidant properties
> - Keep gums strong and prevents and treats gingivitis (a risk factor for cardiovascular disease)
> - Support healthy skin
> - Slow cellular aging.

Dietary sources of CoQ10 include beef heart, pork, chicken liver, mackerel, sardines, walnuts and strawberries, to name a few. Q10 is particularly high in organ meats. With the recommendation that people reduce their consumption of red meat, a natural decline in our consumption of CoQ10 occurs as well. Nevertheless, well over 100 clinical studies at major health institutions have documented CoQ10's heart-protective abilities.

CoQ10 Lowers Blood Pressure

A meta-analysis of human clinical trials using CoQ10 for high blood pressure was led by Professor Frank Rosenfeldt, the Director of the Cardiac Surgical Research Unit at Alfred Hospital in Melbourne, Australia. His team reviewed all published trials of CoQ10 for hypertension and assessed overall efficacy, consistency of therapeutic action, and side-effect incidence. The meta-analysis evaluated 12 clinical trials involving 362 patients comprising three randomized controlled trials, one cross-over study, and eight open-label studies. The research group concluded that coenzyme Q10 has the potential in hypertensive patients to lower systolic blood pressure by up to 17 mm/Hg and diastolic blood pressure by up to 10 mmHg without significant side effects.

Cardiovascular Benefits of CoQ10

■ *Congestive Heart Failure*

CoQ10 in conjunction with standard treatments dramatically improves outcomes in clinical studies of congestive heart failure, which is classified as impairment of the heart's ability to pump enough blood for all of the body's needs. Doses of 300 mg per day improve the heart's ability to pump. CoQ10's antioxidant activity may also contribute to its benefits in treating congestive heart failure.

■ *Stable Angina*

CoQ10 has been studied in humans for stable angina since the early 80s. Angina patients taking 150 mg per day of CoQ10 report a greater ability to exercise without the onset of angina. CoQ10 is also clinically demonstrated to substantially improve arrhythmia and hypertension.

■ *Bad Cholesterol Oxidation*

As mentioned earlier, oxidation of LDL cholesterol in the blood is a key factor in development of cardiovascular disease, and CoQ10 prevents this even more effectively than vitamin E. CoQ10 has also been shown to help reduce the adverse side effects of cardiotoxic chemotherapy drugs, including adriamycin and athralines.

Coenzyme Q10 daily dose: Maintenance dose: 30-100 mg per day with food. Those with congestive heart failure should take 300 mg per day. If you are using statin medications, you need 100-200 mg per day. Those with high blood pressure should take 100-200 mg per day. Or keep it simple by taking 2 capsules of Cala-Q Plus daily with food. Cala-Q Plus contains coenzyme Q10 in the most absorbable form.

♡ An Aspirin a Day?

Aspirin, with its blood-thinning and anti-inflammatory properties, is often recommended to reduce the risk of heart attack reoccurrence. People concerned with heart disease risk are also often counseled to take aspirin preventatively. However, blanket recommendations on the latter point are something the US Preventive Services Task Force attempted to avoid when they came out with their official opinion on aspirin in 2002. Given the knowledge that aspirin increases the incidence of gastrointestinal bleeding and some evidence that aspirin increases the incidence of hemorrhagic stroke, the Task Force suggested that doctors discuss aspirin use only with patients found to be at *high* risk of heart disease (those with a 10-year risk of at least six percent).

A May 2002 article in *The New England Journal of Medicine* took a more moderate stance on aspirin use by concluding that those with a 10-year risk of 15 percent are good candidates for aspirin treatment. Clearly, aspirin use in heart disease is not a cut-and-dried situation. Research continues. Women over the age of 70 should avoid aspirin as it can increase the risk of stroke. For those who have had a heart attack, angioplasty or bypass surgery, a baby aspirin a day can be taken if advised by your physician. Gastrointestinal bleeding is a common side effect of even a baby aspirin per day. In January 2009, the *International Journal of Cardiology* stated that ginger is an effective anti-platelet herb. Drink ginger tea daily, use grated ginger on foods and take ginger capsules as an alternative to baby aspirin.

Marvelous Magnesium

Although magnesium is responsible for over 350 enzymatic functions in the human body, its major role is in the overall health of the heart. As discussed in the Heart-Smart Diet section, magnesium is likened to "nature's calcium channel-blocker" because of its ability to block the entry of calcium into vascular smooth-muscle cells and heart muscle cells. As a result, in addition to eating high-magnesium foods, magnesium supplementation can help lower blood pressure, improve vascular function and aid efficient heart function. Magnesium also helps regulate proper calcium metabolism through its actions on several hormones, including parathyroid hormone and calcitonin in the thyroid.

Potassium and Sodium Need Magnesium

Without magnesium, the cells cannot pump potassium and sodium into and out of the cell. So magnesium deficiency is often the culprit when potassium deficiency is suspected. If you have added potassium to your diet, and still do not see an improvement in heart health, it may be because the potassium is not getting inside the cells where it is needed due to a lack of magnesium.

Magnesium Protects Against Stroke

In one study, 14,221 men and women aged 45–64 years taking part in the first examination of the Atherosclerosis Risk in Communities Study provided blood samples to measure their magnesium levels. Over the course of 15 years of follow-up, the researchers found that blood levels of magnesium were significantly associated with decreased risks of stroke. Specifically, participants taking over 270 mg per day had a 30 percent decreased risk of stroke.

The researchers attributed magnesium's effect on stroke risk reduction to its ability to help maintain healthy blood pressure and to help maintain blood sugar. Magnesium deficiency may be associated with increased inflammation, which increases circulating levels of CRP and triggers cell damage in blood vessel cells.

Magnesium Lowers Bad Cholesterol While Increasing Good Cholesterol

Magnesium works on cholesterol in two ways. One, it regulates enzymes that control the production of cholesterol. Second, it increases levels of good cholesterol HDL while lowering bad cholesterol. Dr. Mildred Seelig, a famous magnesium researcher, says that Lipitor works by inhibiting the production of the HMG CoEnzyme A reductase enzyme that is produced by the liver. This enzyme is also necessary for the production of coenzyme Q10, which is critical for optimal heart health. HMG CoEnzyme A reductase is also converted into another compound known as mevalonate, a fatty acid derivative. Mevalonate is also converted into cholesterol or it can be converted into several plaque-forming substances. Dr. Seelig found that as long as the body has adequate magnesium, it will naturally regulate the HMG CoEnzyme A and cholesterol manufacture will be controlled. But if you become deficient in magnesium, the HMG CoEnzyme A will increase plaque formation in the arteries. Magnesium is key to keeping arteries clear and cholesterol levels healthy.

Magnesium Regulates Blood Pressure

Magnesium supplements have a significant effect on lowering high blood pressure. Japanese researchers have finally clarified inconsistent results from other investigations of magnesium and blood pressure. Some results had indicated that magnesium lowered high blood pressure whereas other research did not. Japanese research following individuals over an eight-week period showed that blood pressure was significantly lower while taking magnesium. And the higher the blood pressure, the larger the decrease seen in those supplementing with magnesium. Researchers believe magnesium acts to relax blood vessels, an effect proven to help lower blood pressure. When blood vessels are constricted – not relaxed – the heart works harder to pump blood through the body, causing blood pressure to increase.

Women should be particularly interested in magnesium supplementation if they have high blood pressure. Often, traditional high blood pressure medications do not work as well for women, but magnesium supplementation works fabulously in women to normalize high blood pressure. High blood pressure medications can cause erectile dysfunction in men. With this in mind, men should be employing natural remedies to reduce high blood pressure as well.

Not All Magnesium Supplements are Created Equal

Magnesium supplements are available in numerous salt forms, as well as bound to amino acids. The absorption rate and tolerability varies greatly between different magnesium supplements. Many are poorly tolerated at therapeutic doses due to this mineral's laxative effect.

Magnesium in its inorganic state (simple salt) is only absorbed at five to 10 percent. Inorganic minerals must be altered from their natural state before they can penetrate the intestinal barrier. The most efficient way to achieve this is by combining them with amino acids. Magnesium joined to the amino acid glycine is the best form because it's best absorbed and is also able to cross the blood brain barrier.

Magnesium glycinate daily dose: Take one to two capsules of Magnesium Bisglycinate daily, providing 200-400 mg of elemental magnesium bisglycinate. Alternatively, mix one scoop of Magsmart in water to taste providing 280 mg of elemental magnesium bisglycinate.

Multivitamins and Minerals to the Rescue

A good multivitamin with minerals is important for preventing heart problems. Multivitamins with minerals contain potassium along with other necessary cofactors for a healthy heart, including B vitamin complex, beta-carotene, vitamins A, C, E as well as the minerals selenium, magnesium and calcium.

Vitamin E improves circulation, has natural gentle blood-thinning properties, reduces oxidized bad cholesterol, and helps prevent heart disease. In a multivitamin with mineral formula, look for a dosage of 200 IU of vitamin E per day. If you are on Coumadin, you can take 200 IU per day but not more.

Beta carotene in dosages of 12,500 IU per day have been shown to protect the heart. Several controversial studies using extremely high doses of beta-carotene and vitamin A, 75,000 IU per day, found it caused adverse effects.

B vitamins and folic acid have been found to lower the risk of heart disease and heart attack. High homocysteine is a risk factor for heart disease because it can cause cholesterol to create plaque formation on the walls of arteries and vessels. B vitamins especially B5, B3, B12 and folic acid can help reduce homocysteine.

Vitamin C, a potent antioxidant, protects blood vessel linings and lowers lipoprotein A (Lp[a]), a type of cholesterol linked to increased risk of heart disease.

It is easier to get these nutrients in a good multivitamin with minerals. Vitamins and minerals are the foundation of your heart smart nutrient program. A recent study into the use of vitamins in relation to mortality found that multivitamins and vitamin E were associated with decreased risks of cardiovascular disease mortality. Always take your multinutrient formula with food.

♡ What Makes a Great Multivitamin with Minerals?

Scientists at Harvard Medical School have advised all adults to take multivitamins with minerals every day to help prevent deficiencies of nutrients that may contribute to a multitude of health problems. Suboptimal levels of folic acid and vitamins B6 and B12, deficient levels of calcium and vitamin D, can all contribute to degenerative disease.

While the market is flooded with multi-nutrient formulas, many contain only the Food and Drug Administration's or Health Canada's recommended dietary allowance (RDAs) of vitamins and minerals. While those amounts may be sufficient to prevent diseases such as scurvy, we know that vibrant health requires nutrients in optimal amounts.

Research also shows that the body more readily uses certain forms of vitamins and minerals than others. Many vitamin combinations on the market today use the cheapest available forms of vitamins and minerals or worse yet, don't label what forms are found in the pill. Make sure you purchase nutrients from a reputable company that manufactures under good manufacturing processes (GMP) and that also third party independently tests their finished nutrients for potency and purity. Make sure the label states the type of nutrient and the quality. Your multinutrient formula should disclose the source of its ingredients. For example, instead of just saying magnesium, the label should say magnesium (as citrate, oxide, chelate, glycinate).

Is your multinutrient formula in capsule form? Most people find capsules easier to digest. Or better yet, does your formula contain betaine hydrochloride to help digest the nutrients? The formula should be designed for your unique needs. If you are a woman, you will need different nutrients than a man.

Multivitamin daily dose: Take 6 capsules of Multismart per day with food or shake one packet of Multismart powder vigorously with water or juice.

Hard Arteries and Vitamin K2

Hardening of the arteries results when excess calcium and fatty substances such as cholesterol and triglycerides accumulate on the wall of the artery, thereby impeding blood flow to and from the heart.

Calcium is an essential mineral used by the body for more than just strong bones. Calcium is needed for the contraction of smooth muscles in the arteries and skeleton among other things. The body keeps calcium in check by removing excess calcium but when calcium metabolism becomes impaired, excess calcium deposits in the arteries and soft tissues (breast and skin).

Calcification of the arteries was once thought to be a normal part of aging and irreversible. But now we know that this process is regulated by vitamin K2. Healthy arterial cells have up to 50 times more vitamin K2 than unhealthy arteries.

Vitamin K1 is known for its ability to maintain normal blood clotting via the liver, whereas vitamin K2 acts to keep arteries healthy. Decades of research has shown that vitamin K2 can reverse stiffness by mobilizing calcium out of arterial cells.

The 10 year Rotterdam Study shows that a high intake of vitamin K2 – but not vitamin K1 – has a strong protective effect on cardiovascular health. This population-based study followed 4807 men and women over age 55 taking vitamin K2 daily. This study found that consuming 32 mcg of vitamin K2 daily resulted in a 50% reduction of arterial calcification, a 50% reduction in death from cardiovascular disease and a 25% reduction in death from all causes. Another study in 2008 following 16,000 women aged 49-70, found that for every 10 mcg of vitamin K2-MK7 consumed the risk of heart disease was reduced by 9%.

Western diets are low in natural vitamin K2. You would have to consume 8 kg of beef, 10 liters of milk or 16 egg yolks to get 100 mcg of vitamin K2-MK7.

Vitamin K2 daily dose: Take one capsule of Bone Booster daily containing vitamin K2-MK7, the superior form of vitamin K2.

Your Heart-Smart Nutrient Program

NUTRIENT	DAILY DOSE
Sytrinol	300 mg with or without food
Pine bark extract	30-200 mg with food
OR Sytrogenol	2 capsules with food
Coenzyme Q10	2 Cala-Q Plus softgels with food
Magnesium	1-2 capsules of Magnesium Bisglycinate with food or mix 1 scoop of Magsmart with water.
Vitamin K2-MK7	1 capsule of Bone Booster with food
Calamari oil	2 Cala-Q Plus softgels with food
Multivitamin with minerals	Take 6 capsules of Multismart with food or shake 1 packet of Multismart powder with water or juice.

ADDITIONAL RECOMMENDATIONS

Drink two to three ounces of pomegranate juice daily.

Drink eight to 10 glasses of pure, filtered water a day or drink herbal tea. Drink before you're thirsty. Thirst is a symptom of dehydration. Store a pitcher of water with lemon slices in the fridge.

Always eat breakfast within half an hour of rising to boost metabolism.

Eat seven to 10 half-cup servings of vegetables daily.

Choose high-quality protein sources no larger than the palm of your hand.

Reduce your consumption of alcohol, table salt and caffeine.

Keep a food journal to help change the way you eat.

Find out what nutrients are depleted by the prescription medications you are taking. An excellent book by Ross Pelton and James LaValle, *The Nutritional Cost of Prescription Drugs*, outlines the reactions of most major types of medications.

Adopt an exercise program like that described in my book *Heart Smart for Women and the Men They Love*.

Seek professionals to provide other beneficial therapies such as chelation therapy, hydrotherapy, acupuncture, massage and traditional Chinese medicine.

chapter nine

How to Tame Stress

Powerful mechanisms like the fight-or-flight response that have evolved through time allow the body to shift into "survival" mode so we can either fight back or escape a perceived threat. In such times of stress, various hormones within the body are secreted to relay orders. In the musculoskeletal system, muscles tense up. The nervous system reconfigures to best preserve and utilize the body's energy stores. Focus is diverted away from unessential areas like the digestive system and diverted towards the heart and brain where adrenaline and noradrenaline speed up our reaction time, heart rate, and blood pressure and increase the blood volume pumped from the heart. The heart starts to pound, breathing quickens and becomes shallow, and we may start to sweat. It is no coincidence that these symptoms match those often found during a heart attack episode. Acute stress has short-term and long-term implications for cardiovascular health. Stress can also trigger anxiety attacks, which are sometimes mistaken for heart attacks.

More stress hormones relay messages to boost sugar, triglyceride and cholesterol levels in the blood. The blood also gets sticky in case we're injured and need to form clots so we're less likely to bleed to death. The immune system responds, ready to protect us. Over the short-term, this hormonal orchestra is designed to perform effectively. Prolonged stress, however, weakens these mechanisms, reducing immunity, causing systemic wear and tear and creating a host of physical, behavioral, emotional and mental symptoms. Although we're probably not trying to fight off a dangerous predator like our ancestors might have been, we're stuck in traffic jams and conference calls. We're cramming our days full of activities and events. And regardless of what kind of stress we're under, self-imposed or otherwise – be it physical, mental, emotional or financial – the body perceives it in the same way. The brain categorizes all stress as deserving a fight-or-flight response and signals hormones to act. Over the course of a normal day, we are activating our stress response repeatedly, and this is where the problems lie.

Take a Stress Test

The following statements determine your happiness level, how you handle stress and if you have negative thinking. Check off the situations that apply to you. Then total the points for the situations you checked off.

☐	I am worried about paying my bills this month.	1
☐	I look at myself in the mirror and think negative thoughts.	3
☐	I am not content with my body.	3
☐	I almost always fake orgasm.	2
☐	I am lonely.	3
☐	I dislike my job.	3
☐	I like my job but have too much work to do.	3
☐	I like my job, but my boss is too demanding.	1
☐	I am always trying to please everyone.	2
☐	I am exhausted but keep going.	3
☐	Sometimes my stomach feels like it has butterflies.	3
☐	I shop to make myself feel better.	1
☐	I have feelings of guilt or anger.	2
☐	I have feelings of inadequacy (not feeling good enough).	3

☐ I am afraid of failure.	2
☐ I have feelings of anxiety or low moods.	2
☐ I feel trapped or that I can't cope sometimes.	3
☐ I crave sugar.	1
☐ I am a single mother/father.	2
☐ I am a university student.	1
☐ I am in an unhappy marriage.	3
☐ I live with an alcoholic or drug abuser.	2
☐ I work shift work.	1
☐ I work too much and don't have enough play time.	1
☐ I get angry with myself.	2
☐ I hold resentment toward my partner.	3
☐ I cannot discuss my sexual desires with my partner.	2
☐ I don't eat regularly (I wait more than four or five hours between meals).	3
☐ I am sick more than three times a year.	1
☐ I lack sexual desire.	1
☐ I smoke.	3
☐ I drink alcohol more than twice a week.	3
☐ I drink too much caffeine.	2
☐ My family and friends are not supportive of the things I do.	2
☐ I am tired all the time.	3
☐ I have friends who take but never give.	2

Your Stress Score

15 or less.
You are handling stress but need to find more balance in your life.

16-30.
You know you have to make some changes fast. You are at risk of exhaustion.

30 or more.
You are highly stressed. You need to adopt strategies to reduce your risk of stress-related disease immediately.

Why We Need to De-stress

Initially, stress can enhance performance, but after a certain point, it causes mental fatigue and the feeling of being overwhelmed. Mental, emotional and physical health suffers. Stress is linked to chest pain, arrhythmia, high blood pressure, stomach problems, sleep disturbances, depression, anger, burnout, overeating, undereating, drug or alcohol abuse, relationship conflicts, social withdrawal and much more. Stress permeates all aspects of life and is inescapable. The trick is to find a healthy balance that enhances good productivity yet includes relaxing regularly. The heart greatly benefits from routine relaxation generated by the following anti-stress strategies.

Deep Breathing for Relaxation

Have you ever considered how you breathe? Do this quick test now. Sit comfortably on a chair. Place one hand on your chest, the other on your belly. Breathe several times. If your chest-bound hand moves more than your belly hand, you are what is known as a thoracic breather; if your belly-bound hand moves more than your chest hand, you're a belly breather. Belly, or diaphragmatic, breathing is what we instinctively did as babies. Besides providing more oxygen to the system, it also allows us to expel more carbon dioxide wastes. Most people expand their chests when they breathe, which elevates the shoulders and is, in fact, a relatively shallow way of inhaling. Better breathing – belly breathing – pushes the abdomen in and out more forcefully, pumping more oxygen into the system.

Tuning in to how you breathe requires mindfulness and practice. Do deep breathing daily, at whatever time and in whatever form suits you. The general rule is, breathe in and out through your nose (not your mouth). Breathe deeply and regularly, eyes closed, with intention and inward focus. Envision your breaths as waves, encroaching and receding, if it helps. Even two or three minutes can make a very beneficial difference.

Yoga: Ancient Practice Has Heart
More than 5,000 years old, yoga unites body, mind and spirit, and also combines elements of relaxation, guided imagery, visualization and meditation. Yoga comes in several forms. "Hatha yoga," which focuses on gentle stretching poses and supportive breathing, is best suited to relaxation purposes and breaking down the muscle patterns of stress. Hatha yoga won't result in the same ultra-sweaty state as power "ashtanga" or hot-room "bikram" yoga, but that's okay when relaxation is your purpose.

Regular yoga improves mood, circulation, digestion, breathing, immunity, flexibility and muscle tone. A recent study including yoga practice for cancer patients confirmed several heart-supportive effects as well. Fifty-nine cancer patients followed an eight-week "mindfulness-based stress reduction" program including relaxation, meditation and gentle yoga that was found to reduce stress symptoms, inflammatory markers, cortisol levels and systolic blood pressure. Conversely, immunity and mood improved. In another study involving 10 patients with cardiovascular disease and 23 without, a six-week program involving yoga and meditation for 90 minutes, three times a week, improved the function of the endothelial cells lining arteries by 69 percent. Regardless of whether the participants had heart disease or not, their blood pressure, resting heart rate and BMI decreased during the study period. Long-term yoga practice (for one year or more) is also associated with increased insulin sensitivity, and has been found to be beneficial for patients with chronic heart failure as a form of exercise that lowered inflammation markers and improved quality of life.

Meditate Stress Away
You don't have to sit on a rock, or be cross-legged and bald, to meditate. The practice of meditation has evolved past old stereotypes into one with applications suited to modern life. We know that depression is one of several psychosocial factors that increases

the risk of heart disease. In 2009, the first large clinical trial investigated the effect of psychosocial intervention on the heart. Two hundred and eight patients with heart failure were followed for a year after eight weeks of training in meditation, coping skills and support group discussion. Compared to a control group, the participants reported lower anxiety and depression, and improved symptoms of heart failure, even at the one year mark.

The combination of meditation and breathing generated positive effects in a recent randomized pilot trial involving 52 patients who didn't receive pharmaceutical treatment for high blood pressure. Those who underwent eight weeks of meditation and breathing techniques "induced clinically relevant and consistent decreases in heart rate, systolic and diastolic blood pressure." A 2006 study noted that yoga with meditation improved endothelial function in people with coronary artery disease, and that this combination resulted in significant reductions in blood pressure, heart rate and BMI in the 33 subjects, whether they had existing heart disease or not. In a randomized, controlled trial of 103 heart disease patients, transcendental meditation for 16 weeks improved blood pressure, insulin resistance and cardiac autonomic nervous system tone compared to a control group receiving health education.

Stress and the Adrenal Connection
The adrenal glands are among the most important glands in the body. These two small glands sit on top of the kidneys and secrete the stress-response hormones including cortisol. Stress hormones are involved in the 'fight or flight' response which tells the body to stay and deal with the stressor or run away.

Adrenal hormones help us deal with stressors such as emotional shocks, infection, high workload, weather changes, environmental chemicals, or physical or emotional trauma. The adrenals also produce the hormones estrogen, testosterone, DHEA and progesterone. The adrenal glands become the back-up hormone system in women when the ovaries take a much needed rest at menopause.

Besides overseeing female transitions, managing the stress response and its corresponding physiological effects in the body like heart rate and breathing rate, and playing a vital role in blood sugar regulation, the adrenals also regulate sodium and water in the body. This balance is crucial to heart health because an improper sodium-potassium ratio contributes to high blood pressure.

Continual exposure to stressors causes excess cortisol to be secreted. If stress is unrelenting the adrenal glands eventually become exhausted to the point where they are no longer able to secrete the necessary hormones. We call this adrenal exhaustion. This is a serious concern because the adrenal glands regulate hundreds of body functions especially cardiovascular health.

Herbs to Reduce Stress

Herbs that assist the body in adapting to stress by supporting the adrenal glands are aptly called adaptogens. Adaptogens have a normalizing effect – regardless of the condition, they help the body maintain the constant internal state necessary for health and life itself. For example, if blood pressure is high, an adaptogen will help lower it; if it is low, the same adaptogen will help normalize it. The best herbs for reducing the effects of stress and supporting heart function are rhodiola, ashwagandha, suma, and schizandra.

■ *Rhodiola (Rhodiola rosea)*

Rhodiola is one of the newer adaptogens to North America, but it has been studied intensively for over 35 years in Russia. Russian researchers have observed that rhodiola increases resistance to a variety of chemical, biological, and physical stressors, as well as offering cardio-protective effects particularly normalizing high blood pressure. It also improves the nervous system and mental function by increasing blood supply. Rhodiola is beneficial in the treatment of insomnia, and enhances mental performance, reduces fatigue and hypertension, improves memory, and relieves depression.

■ *Ashwagandha (Withania somnifera)*
Ashwagandha has been used in Ayurvedic medicine, the traditional medical system of India, for more than 3,000 years. A unique form of ashwagandha, called Sensoril®, has been extensively researched for stress reduction, fatigue, glucose management, cognition, weight loss and improved cardiovascular function. Sensoril Ashwagandha helps combat the negative effects of stress. Sensoril features the highest levels of withanolides – the active ingredient in ashwagandha – which mimic the body's own stress-reducing hormones.

Sensoril has been researched for cardiovascular health. Sensoril's ability to lower stress and cortisol led to significant reductions in blood sugar levels, C-reactive protein, and blood lipids like triglycerides and "bad" LDL cholesterol in human clinical trials. In a double-blind clinical trial over 100 patients, aged 50 to 59 years, took a daily dose of Sensoril. The daily dosage resulted in a decrease in serum cholesterol and there was a significant reduction in the erythrocyte sedimentation rate (ESR). ESR is a measure used to determine inflammation. A high ESR means more pain and inflammation in the body.

■ *Suma (Pfaffia paniculata)*
In Brazil, suma is also called "para todo," a Portuguese phrase meaning "for everything." Traditionally, it is used as an energy and rejuvenation tonic, as well as a general cure-all for many types of disorders. Its active ingredients include phytosterols, beta-sitosterol and stigmasterol, along with glycosides and saponins. Suma is particularly useful in aiding the adrenal glands in times of stress and in treating adrenal fatigue. Suma is an excellent herb for the cardiovascular system. Due to suma's phytosterols it is also used to help normalize high cholesterol.

■ *Schizandra (Schizandra chinensis)*
In traditional Chinese medicine, schizandra is commonly used as a general tonic herb to purify the blood and restore the liver. It counteracts the effects of stress and fatigue. Scientific studies show it has normalizing effects in cases of insomnia, gastrointestinal problems, and immune system disorders. Schizandra improves mental function and enhances physical and intellectual endurance.

Adrenasmart daily dose: Take Adrenasmart, an adaptogenic formula containing rhodiola, Sensoril® ashwagandha, suma, and schizandra. For optimal results take 1 to 2 capsules of Adrenasmart at 3:00 in the afternoon with a protein snack when you feel a drop in energy.

Do You Live with Heart?
It is hopefully clear by now that the heart is more than just an organ with a job to do. Sometimes, in the rush of modern life as we're racing to work, to meet friends, to catch a plane, to make it to the video store before closing, to meet a deadline, we forget this fact. Everybody, even the most enlightened, needs the occasional reminder about the need to nurture our inner selves. "Living with heart" not only cultivates happiness, balance, passion and a more positive outlook, but it also sends powerful cellular messages that impact physical health.

Positive thoughts generate good moods, which initiate healthy decisions and physical effects. Conversely, negative thoughts contribute to and exacerbate dark moods, which can lead to unhealthy behaviors and symptoms of stress with further health implications. So how do we break patterns of negativity and set ourselves on the positive path? By retraining our thoughts, just as we can retrain our patterns of eating, exercising, sitting, sleeping, breathing and driving. There are many excellent books available on this subject.

Laughter: The Best Medicine?

Have you ever gone to a movie and come out with your stomach aching from having laughed so hard? What an amazing feeling. You were also probably happy, talkative, bubbling with energy. It likely wasn't a conscious choice to be in a good mood; you simply couldn't help yourself. Laughter and smiling reduce the symptoms of depression, physical and emotional pain, and shared laughter creates relationships. When we laugh, the body releases endorphins. These "feel-good" hormones are natural painkillers and bring about the slight euphoria that also accompanies a good workout. Laughter relieves stress hormones, improves immunity, lowers inflammation in the body and even affects blood sugar levels. Research has found that the endothelial cells in the inner arteries have receptors that attract the endorphins generated by laughter. This joining leads to the direct release of nitrous oxide, which relaxes muscles and results in vessel dilation.

Visit your local DVD rental store. Stock up on comedies, sitcoms and Disney and Pixar classics. (They're not just for kids.)

Humor-ize your screensaver. Search Google images for funny pictures, raid your photo albums, or hit your favorite cartoon website.

Post laugh reminders. Make a point of reading the comics in your local paper. Clip out any good ones and post them on your fridge or on your bathroom mirror.

Join a laughter club or try laughter yoga. Yes, there is actually a non-profit group that facilitates the latter. The website www.laughteryoga.org has an exercise routine that "provides an excellent cardiovascular workout and heart massage."

Self-honesty: Emotions and Expression

In earlier sections, you have seen how negative emotions are linked to heart disease. Anger, hostility, anxiety and depression can worsen cardiovascular troubles. Likewise, when a diagnosis of heart disease is given, it's common to feel shocked, upset or depressed. However, strong support from those around you and a multidimensional plan like the one explained in this book can help move you into the next stage: acceptance. Here is where another component of true heart healing – emotional and psychological – lies. Acceptance sets the stage for emotional honesty, which helps us regain/ find our sense of self and our purpose in life.

We must learn to listen and accept any inward-derived messages. Are we being emotionally honest with ourselves? Pretend your heart is your best friend; what would your best friend want to say to you? Of course, this level of self-reflection is not always easy. The issues that come to light might be small (e.g., forgiving a grievance against an ex-coworker) or large (e.g., dealing with issues of abuse or family trauma). Some people will be able to do this alone, some will need guidance. Whichever way works best for you is acceptable.

As we become more emotionally and mentally conscious, we are happier, less stressed and less prone to anxiety and depression. We are more engaged in life. Naturally, communication is a key factor in this transformation. We must learn to be honest with not only ourselves but also with the people in our lives – our partners, siblings, friends, colleagues and acquaintances.

Other Important Heart-Smart Tips

■ *Get a pet.* Animals help us relax, lower blood pressure, enhance emotions and help us deal with change and loss.

■ **Phone a friend.** Regular interaction with people who care is essential to a well-balanced life. Loneliness is a major predictor of disease.

■ **Build your support team.** This means some combination of a spouse, family and friends but can also include a support group, religious group, hobby group, and/or various health-care professionals.

■ **Share how you feel and think.** If you have been recently diagnosed with heart disease or its risk factors, the people in your life are going through it as well. Talk with them, share your resources. They may want to help but don't know how. Ask them for what you need support-wise, but it's okay to draw boundaries if you need personal time or if they're overzealous in expressing their opinions of what you should do. Remember, it's your health journey.

■ **Find joy in play.** Rediscover your inner child. Lightheartedness enhances immunity, and increases creativity and cheer in all aspects of our lives.

■ **Be grateful.** Before bed each night, express what you're grateful for in your life. People who perform daily gratitude exercises are more alert, enthusiastic, determined and optimistic. Grateful people also report having fewer physical complaints and more energy.

■ **Give of yourself.** By focusing outward, you attract abundance. Directing attention away from yourself benefits others and allows you to take a realistic look at how lucky you are. Altruism and compassion deactivate negative emotions that affect your immune, hormone and cardiovascular systems.

■ **Start a journal.** Writing is a great form of self-expression. Better to write out what you're feeling than to repress it or express it unhealthfully. Writing helps recovery after trauma/emotional upset and also improves health by bolstering certain immune factors.

■ **Listen to music.** Music therapy is a wonderful wellness tool. Play a CD or listen to the radio while you get ready for work, commute, cook, eat, clean or prepare for bed. Experiment with song writing, performing, developing lyrics. Join a music appreciation club and attend live productions.

■ **Take a nap.** This simple pleasure can improve cardiac health. A daily half-hour mid-day nap cuts heart attack risk by 30 percent. A one-hour nap, by 50 percent.

■ **Have sex.** The intimacy that sensuality and sexuality generate profoundly influences well-being. If you had a heart attack, check with your doctor about when to resume having sex. It's usually within a few weeks. The physical exertion of normal sexual activity is within the range of routine daily activities like brisk walking, golf or carrying a full bag of groceries. Still, a reintroduction to sex shouldn't be rushed. Interestingly, regular exercise after a heart attack practically eliminates the risk of a reoccurrence during sex. The more you exercise (including having sex), the lower your risk.

References and Resources

Introduction

American Heart Foundation, Heart Disease and Stroke Statistics, 2009 Update At-a-Glance, www.americanheart.org

Heart and Stroke Foundation of Canada, Website Statistics, www.heartandstroke.com

All About the Heart

Herron K et al. "High intake of cholesterol results in less atherogenic low-density lipoprotein particles in men and women independent of response classification*1." Metabolism, 2004; 53(6): 823-830.

Harman NL, Leeds AR, Griffin BA. "Increased dietary cholesterol does not increase plasma low density lipoprotein when accompanied by an energy-restricted diet and weight loss." Eur J Nutr, 2008 Oct; 47(1): 408.

Iglay HB et al. "Moderately increased protein intake predominately from egg sources does not influence whole body, regional, or muscle composition responses to resistance training in older people." J Nutr Health Aging. 2009 Feb; 13(2): 108-14.

Heart Disease Risks

Kirsten Bibbins-Domingo, PhD, et al. "Adolescent Overweight and Future Adult Coronary Heart Disease." NEJM. 2007 Dec 6; 357(23): 2371-2379.

Visser, M, PhD, et al. "Elevated C-Reactive Protein Levels in Overweight and Obese Adults." JAMA. 1999; 282: 2131-2135.

Yusuf S, et al. "Obesity and the risk of myocardial infarction in 27,000 participants from 52 countries, a case-controlled study." Lancet 2005; 366: 1640-1649.

Piepoli MF, et al. "Exercise training meta-analysis of trials in patients with chronic heart failure (ExTraMATCH)." BMJ. 2004 Jan 24; 328(7433): 189. Epub 2004 Jan 16.

Passino C et al. "Aerobic Training Decreases B-Type Natriuretic Peptide Expression and Adrenergic Activation in Patients With Heart Failure" Journal of the American College of Cardiology. 2006; 47(9): 1835-1839.

The Lowdown on Cholesterol and Blood Pressure

National Heart, Lung and Blood Institute's National Cholesterol Education Program Cholesterol Level Recommendations, 2001

Xilin Y, et al. "Independent Associations Between Low-density Lipoprotein Cholesterol and Cancer Among Patients with Type 2 Diabetes Mellitus." CMAJ. 2008 August; 179(5): 427-37.

Sachdeva A, et al. "Lipid Levels in Patients Hospitalized with Coronary Artery Disease: An Analysis of 136,905 Hospitalizations in Get With The Guidelines." Am Heart J. 2009 Jan; 157(1): 111-117.e2.

Recommended Triglyceride Levels for the US and Canada, The Mayo Clinic, www.mayoclinic.com

Danesh J, et al. "Lipoprotein(a) and Coronary Heart Disease" Circulation. 2000; 102: 1082

Lipoprotein A and Apolipoprotein B Levels, US National Institutes of Health, Medline Plus (for the US) www.nlm.nih.gov/medlineplus/ and (for Canada) Jacques Genest J, et al. "Recommendations for the Management of Dyslipidemia and the Prevention of Cardiovascular Disease: 2003 Update." CMAJ. 2003; 168(9): 921-4.

Whincup P, et al. "Serum total homocysteine and coronary heart disease: prospective study in middle aged men." Heart. 1999 October; 82(4): 448–454.

Graham IM, FRCPI, et al. "Plasma Homocysteine as a Risk Factor for Vascular Disease." JAMA. 1997, June 11; 277(22): 1775-1781.

Malinow MR, et al. "Homocyst(e)ine, Diet, and Cardiovascular Diseases: A Statement for Healthcare Professionals from the Nutrition Committee, American Heart Association." Circulation. 1999; 99: 178-82.

Metamatrix Clinical Laboratories Cardiovascular Health Profile Testing, used by Naturopathic Doctors http://www.metametrix.com/DirectoryOfServices/pdf/pdf_sample_0161 CardiovascularHealth-Blood.pdf

Robinson K, et al. "Hyperhomocysteinemia and Low Pyridoxal Phosphate. Common and Independent Reversible Risk Factors for Coronary Artery Disease." Circulation. 1995 Nov 15; 92(10): 2825-30.

Ferritin Testing Ranges – US National Institutes of Health Medline Plus, www.nlm.nih.gov/medlineplus/

Coppola G, et al. "Fibrinogen as a predictor of mortality after acute myocardial infarction: a forty-two-month follow-up study." Ital Heart J. 2005 Apr; 6(4): 315-22.

Zoccali C, et al. "Fibrinogen, mortality and incident cardiovascular complications in end-stage renal failure." J Intern Med. 2003 Aug; 254(2): 132-9.

Aono Y, et al. "Plasma Fibrinogen, Ambulatory Blood Pressure, and Silent Cerebrovascular Lesions: The Ohasama Study." Arterioscler Thromb Vasc Biol. 2007 Apr; 27(4): 963-8.

Fibrinogen Studies Collaboration, Danesh J, et al. "Plasma Fibrinogen Level and the Risk of Major Cardiovascular Diseases and Nonvascular Mortality: An Individual Participant Meta-analysis." JAMA. 2005 Oct 12; 294(14): 1799-809.

Fibrinogen Testing Ranges – US National Institutes of Health Medline Plus, www.nlm.nih.gov/medlineplus/

Optimal Fibrinogen Levels – Life Extension Foundation, www.lef.org

Ridker PM, et al. 'Inflammation, Aspirin, and the Risk of Cardiovascular Disease in Apparently Healthy Men." N Engl J Med. 1997 Apr 3; 336(14): 973-9.

Ridker PM, et al. "Prospective Study of C-reactive Protein and the Risk of Future Cardiovascular Events Among Apparently Healthy Women." Circulation. 1998 Aug 25; 98(8): 731-3.

American Blood Pressure Statistics, American Heart Foundation, www.americanheart.org

Canadian Blood Pressure Statistics, the Heart and Stroke Foundation of Canada, www.heartandstroke.com

Diabetes and Depression: Double Trouble

Centers for Disease Control, National Diabetes Fact Sheet 2007, www.cdc.gov/diabetes/pubs/pdf/ndfs_2007.pdf

Diabetes-Heart Disease Connection, American Diabetes Association, www.diabetes.org/heart-disease-stroke.jsp

Khaw K, et al. "Glycated Haemoglobin, Diabetes, and Mortality in Men in Norfolk Cohort of European Prospective Investigation of Cancer and Nutrition (EPIC-Norfolk)." BMJ 2001 (6 January); 322: 15.

Glucose Tolerance Testing, National Institutes of Health Medline Plus, www.nlm.nih.gov/medlineplus/ency/article/003466.htm

Diabetes Prevention Program Research Group. "Reduction in the Incidence of Type 2 Diabetes with Lifestyle Intervention or Metformin." NEJM. 2002 February 7; 346(6): 393-403.

Ratner RE, et al. "Prevention of Diabetes in Women with a History of Gestational Diabetes: Effects of Metformin and Lifestyle Interventions." The Journal of Clinical Endocrinology & Metabolism. 2008; 93(12): 4774-4779.

The Diabetes Prevention Program Research Group. "Effect of Progression From Impaired Glucose Tolerance to Diabetes on Cardiovascular Risk Factors and Its Amelioration by Lifestyle and Metformin Intervention" Diabetes Care. 2009 April; 32(4): 726-732

Depression Symptoms, the College of Family Physicians of Canada, www.cfpa.ca

McGrath, E et al. "Women and Depression: Risk Factors and Treatment Issues." 1990. Washington, DC: American Psychological Association.

Penninx BW, et al. "Depression and Cardiac Mortality: Results from a Community-based Longitudinal Study." Arch Gen Psychiatry. 2001 Mar; 58(3): 221-7.

Whang W, et al. "Depression and Risk of Sudden Cardiac Death and Coronary Heart Disease in Women." J Am Coll Cardiol. 2009; 53: 950-958.

Wellenius GA, et al. "Depressive Symptoms and the Risk of Atherosclerotic Progression Among Patients With Coronary Artery Bypass Grafts." Circulation. 2008; 117: 2313-2319.

Reed D, et al. "Social Networks and Coronary Heart Disease among Japanese Men in Hawaii." Am J Epidemiol. 1983 Apr; 117(4):384-96.

Bunker SJ, et al. " 'Stress' and Coronary Heart Disease: Psychosocial Risk Factors." Med J Aust. 2003 Mar 17; 178(6): 272-6.

"Can Pets Help Keep You Healthy? Exploring the Human-Animal Bond" NIH News in Health, National Institutes of Health, February 2009, eNewsletter.

Mittleman MA, MDCM, DrPH, et al. "Triggering of Acute Myocardial Infarction Onset by Episodes of Anger." Circulation. 1995; 92: 1720-1725.

Yoichi C, MD, PhD and Steptoe A, DPhil. "The Association of Anger and Hostility with Future Coronary Heart Disease: A Meta-Analytic Review of Prospective Evidence." J Am Coll Cardiol. 2009; 53: 936-946.

The Heart-Smart Diet

Assuncao ML, et al. "Effects of Dietary Coconut Oil on the Biochemical and Anthropometric Profiles of Women Presenting Abdominal Obesity." Lipids. 2009 May 13; [Epub ahead of print].

Vesselinovitch D, et al. "Atherosclerosis in the Rhesus Monkey Fed Three Food Fats." Atherosclerosis. 1974 Sep-Oct; 20(2): 303-21.

Oh K, et al. "Dietary Fat Intake and Risk of Coronary Heart Disease in Women: 20 Years of Follow-up of the Nurses' Health Study." Am J Epidemiol. 2005; 161(7): 672-679.

Shekelle RB, et al. "Diet, Serum Cholesterol, and Death from Coronary Heart Disease. The Western Electric Study." NEJM. 1981; 304(2): 65-70.

Oh K, et al. "Dietary Fat Intake and Risk of Coronary Heart Disease in Women: 20 Years of Follow-up of the Nurses' Health Study." Am J Epidemiol. 2005; 161(7): 672-679.

Ascherio A, et al. "Dietary Fat and Risk of Coronary Heart Disease in Men: Cohort Follow up Study in the United States." BMJ. 1996; 313(7049): 84-90.

Laaksonen DE, et al. "Prediction of Cardiovascular Mortality in Middle-aged Men by Dietary and Serum Linoleic and Polyunsaturated Fatty Acids." Arch Intern Med. 2005; 165(2): 193-199.

Stone NJ. "Fish Consumption, Fish Oil, Lipids, and Coronary Heart Disease." Circulation. 1996; 94: 2337-2340.

Hu FB, et al. "Fish and Omega-3 Fatty Acid Intake and Risk of Coronary Heart Disease in Women." JAMA. 2002; 287: 1815–1821.

Siscovick DS, et al. "Dietary Intake and Cell Membrane Levels of Long-chain n-3 Polyunsaturated Fatty Acids and the Risk of Primary Cardiac Arrest." JAMA. 1995; 274: 1363–1367

Gillum RF, et al. "The Relationship Between Fish Consumption and Stroke Incidence: The NHANES I Epidemiologic Follow-up Study (National Health and Nutrition Examination Survey). Arch Intern Med. 1996; 156: 537–542.

Iso H, et al. "Intake of Fish and Omega-3 Fatty Acids and Risk of Stroke in Women." JAMA. 2001; 285: 304–312.

Mozaffarian D. "Fish and n-3 Fatty Acids for the Prevention of Fatal Coronary Heart Disease and Sudden Cardiac Death." Am J Clin Nutr. 2008; 87(6): 1991S-1996S.

Sircus, M, OMD. Magnesium: The Ultimate Heart Medicine. eBook, 2009. www.imva.info

Bemelmans WJ, et al. "Increased Alpha-linolenic Acid Intake Lowers C-Reactive Protein But Has No Effect on Markers of Atherosclerosis." Eur J Clin Nutr. 2004; 58(7): 1083-1089.

Rallidis LS, et al. "Dietary Alpha-linolenic Acid Decreases C-reactive Protein, Serum Amyloid A and Interleukin-6 in Dyslipidaemic Patients." Atherosclerosis. 2003; 167(2): 237-242.

Zhao G, et al. "Dietary Alpha-linolenic Acid Reduces Inflammatory and Lipic Cardiovascular Risk Factors in Hypercholesterolemic Men and Women." J Nutr. 2004; 134(11): 2991-2997.

Djousse L, et al. "Relation Between Dietary Linolenic acid and Coronary Artery Disease in the National Heart, Lung and Blood Institute Family Heart Study. Am J Clin Nutr. 2001; 74: 612-619.

James MJ, et al. "Metabolism of Stearidonic Acid in Human Subjects: Comparison with the Metabolism of Other n-3 Fatty Acids." Am J Clin Nutr. 2003 May; 77(5): 1140-5.

Johnson EJ, and Schaefer EJ. "Potential Role of Dietary n–3 Fatty Acids in the Prevention of Dementia and Macular Degeneration." Am J Clin Nutr. 2006; 83(6): S1494-1498S.

Kelly DS, et al. "DHA Supplementation Decreases Serum C-Reactive Protein and Other Markers of Inflammation in Hypertriglyceridemic Men." J Nutr. 2009 Mar; 139(3): 495-501.

Wood, M. "DHA Lowers Blood Triglycerides in Diet Study." Agricultural Research.1999 Sept; 46(9): 18.

Mori TA, et al. "Docosahexaenoic Acid but Not Eicosapentaenoic Acid Lowers Ambulatory Blood Pressure and Heart Rate in Humans." Hypertension. 1999; 34: 253-260. Meyer BJ, et al. "Dose-Dependent Effects of Docosahexaenoic Acid Supplementation on Blood Lipids in Statin-Treated Hyperlipidaemic Subjects." Lipids. 2007; 42(2): 109-15.

Schaefer EJ, et al. "Plasma Phosphatidylcholine Docosahexaenoic Acid Content and Risk of Dementia and Alzheimer Disease: The Framingham Heart Study." Arch Neurol. 2006;63(11): 1545-1550.

Holub BJ. "Docosahexaenoic Acid (DHA) and Cardiovascular Disease Risk Factors." Prostaglandins Leukot Essent Fatty Acids. 2009 Jun 20. [Epub ahead of print].

Halton TL, et al. "Low-carbohydrate-diet score and the risk of coronary heart disease in women." NEJM. 2006; 355(19): 1991-2002.

Sinha R, et al. "Meat Intake and Mortality: A Prospective Study of Over Half a Million People." Arch Intern Med. 2009; 169: 562-571.

Sanchez-Tainta A, et al. "Adherence to a Mediterranean-type Diet and Reduced Prevalence of Clustered Cardiovascular Risk Factors in a Cohort of 3204 High-risk Patients." Eur J Cardiovasc Prev Rehabil. 2008; 15(5): 589-593.

Fito M, et al. "Effect of a Traditional Mediterranean Diet on Lipoprotein Oxidation: A Randomized Controlled Trial." Arch Intern Med. 2007; 167(11): 1195-1203.

Nunez-Cordoba JM, et al. "The Mediterranean Diet and Incidence of Hypertension: The Seguimiento Universidad de Navarra (SUN) Study." Am J Epidemiol. 2009; 169(3): 339-46.

Tortosa A, et al. "Mediterranean Diet Inversely Associated with the Incidence of Metabolic Syndrome: The SUN Prospective Cohort." Diabetes Care. 2007; 30(11): 2957-2959.

Salas-Salvado J, et al. "Effect of a Mediterranean Diet Supplemented With Nuts on Metabolic Syndrome Status: One-Year Results of the PREDIMED Randomized Trial." Arch Intern Med. 2008; 168(22): 2449-2458.

Dedoussis GV, et al. "Mediterranean Diet and Plasma Concentration of Inflammatory Markers in Old and Very Old Subjects in the ZINCAGE Population Study." Clin Chem Lab Med. 2008 May 21.

Kaplan M, et al. "Pomegranate Juice Supplementation to Atherosclerotic Mice Reduces Macrophage Lipid Peroxidation, Cellular Cholesterol Accumulation and Development of Atherosclerosis." Biochemical and Molecular Action of Nutrients. 2001 Aug; 131(8): 2082-9.

Aviram M, et al. "Pomegranate Juice Flavonoids Inhibit Low-density Lipoprotein Oxidation and Cardiovascular Diseases: Studies in Atherosclerotic Mice and Humans. Drugs Under Experimental and Clinical Research. 2002; XXVIII(2-3): 49-62.

Fuhrman B, et al. "Pomegranate Juice Inhibits Oxidized LDL Uptake and Cholesterol Biosynthesis in Macrophages." J Nutr Biochem. 2005 Sep; 16(9): 570-6.

Sumner MD, et al. "Effects of Pomegranate Juice Consumption on Myocardial Perfusion in Patients with Coronary Heart Disease." Am J Cardiol. 2005 Sep 15; 96(6): 810-4.

Aviram M, et al. "Pomegranate Juice Consumption for 3 Years by Patients with Carotid Artery Stenosis Reduces Common Carotid Intima-media Thickness, Blood Pressure and LDL Oxidation." Clin Nutr. 2004 Jun; 23(3): 423-33.

Sastravaha G, et al. "Adjunctive Periodontal Treatment with Centella asiatica and Punica granatum Extracts in Supportive Periodontal Therapy. J Int Acad Periodontol. 2005 Jul; 7(3):70-9.

Huang TH, et al. "Anti-diabetic Action of Punica Granatum Flower Extract: Activation of PPAR-gamma and Identification of an Active Component. Toxicol Appl Pharmacol. 2005 Sep 1; 207(2): 160-9.

Rosenblat M, et al. "Anti-oxidative Effects of Pomegranate Juice (PJ) Consumption by Diabetic Patients on Serum and on Macrophages." Atherosclerosis. 2006 Aug; 187(2): 363-71.

Fung TT, et al. "Sweetened Beverage Consumption and Risk of Coronary Heart Disease in Women." Am J Clin Nutr. 2009; 89(4): 1037-42.

Debette S, et al. "Tea Consumption Is Inversely Associated With Carotid Plaques in Women." Atheroslcerosis, Thrombosis, and Vascular Biology. 2008; 28(2): 353-359.

Gardner EJ, et al. "Black tea--helpful or harmful? A Review of the Evidence." European Journal of Clinical Nutrition. 2007; 61(1): 3-18.

Mozaffari-Khosravi H, et al. "The Effects of Sour Tea (Hibiscus Sabdariffa) on Hypertension in Patients with Type II Diabetes." J Hum Hypertens. 2009 Jan; 23(1): 48-54.

Sacks FM, et al. "Effects on Blood Pressure of Reduced Dietary Sodium and the Dietary Approaches to Stop Hypertension (DASH) Diet. DASH-Sodium Collaborative Research Group." N Engl J Med. 2001 Jan 4; 344(1): 3-10.

Umesawa M, et al. "Sodium, Potassium, Diet Reference: "Relations Between Dietary Sodium and Potassium Intakes and Mortality from Cardiovascular Disease: The Japan Collaborative Cohort Study for Evaluation of Cancer Risks." Am J Clin Nutr. 2008; 88(1): 195-202.

Rosanoff A, and Seelig MS. "Comparison of Mechanism and Functional Effects of Magnesium and Statin Pharmaceuticals." J Am Coll Nutr. 2004; 23(5): 501S-505S.

Almoznino-Sarafian D, et al. "Magnesium Administration May Improve Heart Rate Variability in Patients with Heart Failure." Nutr Metab Cardiovasc Dis. 2009 Feb 6; [Epub ahead of print].

Sepura OB, and Martynow AI. "Magnesium Orotate in Severe Congestive Heart Failure (MACH)." Int J Cardiol. 2009; 134(1): 145-7.

Almoznino-Sarafian D, et al. "Magnesium and C-reactive Protein in Heart Failure: An Anti-inflammatory Effect of Magnesium Administration?" Eur J Nutr. 2007; 46(4): 230-237.

Shechter M, et al. "Effects of Oral Magnesium Therapy on Exercise Tolerance, Exercise-Induced Chest Pain, and Quality of Life in Patients with Coronary Artery Disease." Am J Cardiol. 2003 March 1; 91: 517-521.

Shechter M, et al. "Magnesium Therapy in Acute Myocardial Infarction When Patients Are not Candidates for Thrombolytic Therapy." American Journal of Cardiology. 1995 February 15; 75(5): 321-323.

Miller S, et al. "Effects of Magnesium on Atrial Fibrillation After Cardiac Surgery: A Meta-Analysis." Heart. 2005; 91: 618-623.

Heart-Smart Nutrients

Quereshi A, et al. "Response of Hypercholesterolemic Subjects to Administration of Tocotrienols. Lipid. 1995; 30: 1171-1177.

Talbott SM, et al. "Effect of Citrus Flavonoids and Tocotrienols on Serum Cholesterol Levels in Hypercholesterolemic Subjects." Series of studies submitted to Alternative Therapies in Health and Medicine, Boulder CO.

Araghi-Niknam M, et al. "Pine Bark Extract Reduces Platelet Aggregation." Integr Med. 2000; 2(2): 73-77.

Belcaro G, et al. "Prevention of Venous Thrombophlebitis in Long-haul Flights with Pycnogenol." Clin Appl Thromb Hemost. 2004; 10(4): 373-377.

Buz'Zard AR, et al. "Kyolic and Pycnogenol Increases Human Growth Hormone Secretion in Genetically-engineered Keratinocytes." Growth Hormone & IGF Research. 2002; 12: 34-40.

Cesarone MR, et al. "Prevention of Edema in Long Flights with Pycnogenol." Clin Appl Thromb Hemost. 2005; 11(3): 289-294.

Fitzpatrick DF, et al. "Endothelium-dependent Vascular Effects of Pycnogenol." J Cardiovasc Pharmacol. 1998; 32: 509-515.

Gulati OP. "Pycnogenol in Venous Disorders: A Review." Eur Bull Drug Res. 1999; 7(2): 8-13.

Hasegawa N. "Stimulation of Lipolysis by Pycnogenol." Phytother Res. 1999; 13(7), 619-620.

Hasegawa N. "Inhibition of Lipogenesis by Pycnogenol." Phytother Res. 2000; 14(6): 472-473.

Hosseini SL, et al. "A Randomized, Double-blind, Placebo-controlled, Prospective, 16-week Crossover Study to Determine the Role of Pycnogenol in Modifying Blood Pressure in Mildly Hypertensive Patients." Nutr Res. 2001; 21(9): 67-76.

Hosseini S, et al. "Pycnogenol in the Management of Asthma." Journal of Medicinal Food. 2001b; 4(4): 201-209.

Kohana T, and Suzuki N. "The Treatment of Gynaecological Disorders with Pycnogenol." Eur Bull Drug Res. 1999; 7: 30-32.

Liu X, et al. "Pycnogenol, French Maritime Pine Bark Extract, Improves Endothelial Function of Hypertensive Patients." Life Sci. 2004a; 74(7): 855-862.

Liu X, et al. "Antidiabetic Effect of Pycnogenol French Maritime Pine Bark Extract in Patients with Diabetes Type II." Life Sci. 2004b; 75(21): 2505-2513.

Mochizuki M and Hasegawa N. "Pycnogenol Stimulates Lipolysis in 3t3-L1 Cells Via Stimulation of Beta-receptor Mediated Activity. Phytother Res. 2004; 18(12): 1029-1030.

Nelson AB, et al. "Pycnogenol Inhibits Macrophage Oxidative Burst, Lipoprotein Oxidation, and Hydroxyl Radical-induced DNA Damage." Drug Dev Ind Pharm. 1998; 24(2); 139-144.

Peng Q, et al. "Pycnogenol Inhibits Tumor Necrosis Factor-alpha-induced Nuclear Factor Kappa B Activation and Adhesion Molecule Expression in Human Vascular Endothelial Cells." Cell Mol Life Sci. 2000; 57(5); 834-841.

Packer L, et al. "Antioxidant Activity and Biologic Properties of a Procyanidin-rich Extract from Pine (Pinus maritima) Bark, Pycnogenol." Free Radical Biology and Medicine. 1999; 27(5/6): 704-724.

Pavlovic P. "Improved Endurance by Use of Antioxidants." Eur Bull Drug Res. 1999; 7(2): 26-29.

Putter M, et al. "Inhibition of Smoking-induced Platelet Aggregation by Aspirin and Pycnogenol." Thromb Res. 1999; 95(4): 155-161.

Roseff SJ. "Improvement in Sperm Quality and Function with French Maritime Pine Tree Bark Extract." J Reprod Med. 2002; 47(10): 821-824.

Rihn B, et al. "From Ancient Remedies to Modern Therapeutics: Pine Bark Uses in Skin Disorders Revisited. Phytother Res. 2001; 15: 76-78.

Saliou C, et al. "Solar Ultraviolet-induced Erythema in Human Skin and Nuclear Factor-kappa-B-dependent Gene Expression in Keratinocytes are Modulated by a French Maritime Pine Bark Extract." Free Rad Biol Med. 2001; 30(2): 154-160.

Simme S, and Reeve VE. "Protection from Inflammation, Immunosuppression and Carcinogenesis Induced by UV Radiation in Mice by Topical Pycnogenol." Photochem Photobiol. 2004; 79(2): 193-198.

Tixier JM, et al. "Evidence by In-vivo and In-vitro Studies that Binding of Pycnogenol to Elastin Affects its Rate of Degradation by Elastase." Biochem Pharmacol. 1984; 33: 3933-3939.

Vina J, et al. "Free Radicals in Exhaustive Physical Exercise: Mechanism of Production and Protection by Antioxidants. Life. 2000; 50(4-5): 271-277.

Wei Z, et al. "Pycnogenol Enhances Endothelial Cell Antioxidant Defences." Redox Rep. 1997; 3: 147-155.

Cupp MJ, and Tracy TS, ed. "Chapter 4: Coenzyme Q10 (Ubiquinone, Ubidecarenone)" Dietary Supplements, Humana Press; Totowa (New Jersey), 2003, p. 53-85.

Rosenfeldt FL, et al. "Coenzyme Q10 in the Treatment of Hypertension: A Meta-analysis of the Clinical Trials." J Human Hypertension. 2007; 21: 297-306.

Ohira T. "Serum and Dietary Magnesium and Risk of Ischemic Stroke: The Atherosclerosis Risk in Communities Study." American Journal of Epidemiology Advance Access published on April 16, 2009.

Pocobelli G, et al. "Use of Supplements of Multivitamins, Vitamin C and Vitamin E in Relation to Mortality." Am J Epidemiol. 2009 Aug 15; 170(4): 472-83. Epub 2009 Jul 13.

Dilman V and Dean W. The Neuroendocrine Theory of Aging and Degenerative Disease, The Center for Bio-Gerontology, Pensacola, 1992.

Geleijnse JM, et al. "Dietary Intake of Menaquinone is Associated with a Reduced Risk of Coronary Heart Disease: The Rotterdam Study." J Nutr. 2004 Nov;134(11): 3100-5.

Gast GC, et al. "A High Menaquinone Intake Reduces the Incidence of Coronary Heart Disease." Nutr Metab Cardiovasc Dis. 2009;19: 504-10.

How to Tame Stress

Carlson LE, et al. "One Year Pre-post Intervention Follow-up of Psychological, Immune, Endocrine and Blood Pressure Outcomes of Mindfulness-based Stress Reduction (MBSR) in Breast and Prostate Cancer Outpatients." Brain Behav Immun. 2007 Nov; 21(8): 1038-49.

Jancin B. "Yoga Helps Endothelial Function in Heart Patients." Family Practice News. 2004 December 15: 12.

Chaya MS, et al. "Insulin Sensitivity and Cardiac Autonomic Function in Young Male Practitioners of Yoga." Natl Med J India. 2008 Sep-Oct; 21(5): 217-21.

Pullen PR, et al. "Effects of Yoga on Inflammation and Exercise Capacity in Patients with Chronic Heart Failure." J Card Fail. 2008 Jun; 14(5): 407-13.

Sullivan MJ, et al. "The Support, Education, and Research in Chronic Heart Failure Study (SEARCH): A Mindfulness-based Psychoeducational Intervention Improves Depression and Clinical Symptoms in Patients with Chronic Heart Failure." Am Heart J. 2009 Jan; 157(1): 84-90.

Manikonda JP, et al. "Contemplative Meditation Reduces Ambulatory Blood Pressure and Stress-induced Hypertension: A Randomized Pilot Trial." J Hum Hypertens. 2008 Feb; 22(2): 138-40.

Sivasankaran S. "The Effect of a Six-week Program of Yoga and Meditation on Brachial Artery Reactivity: Do Psychosocial Interventions Affect Vascular Tone?" Clin Cardiol. 2006 Sep; 29(9): 393-8.

Paul-Labrador M, et al. "Effects of a Randomized Controlled Trial of Transcendental Meditation on Components of the Metabolic Syndrome in Subjects with Coronary Heart Disease." Arch Intern Med. 2006 Jun 12; 166(11): 1218-24.

Archana R, and Namasivayam A. "Antistress Effect of Withania Somnifera." J Ethnopharmacol. 1999 Jan; 64(1): 91-3.

Bhattacharya SK, and Muruganandam AV. "Adaptogenic Activity of Withania Somnifera: An Experimental Study Using a Rat Model of Chronic Stress." Pharmacol Biochem Behav. 2003 Jun; 75(3): 547-55.

Bone K. Clinical Applications of Ayurvedic and Chinese Herbs. Monographs for the Western Herbal Practitioner. Australia: Phytotherapy Press, 1996:137-141.

Shevtsov VA, et al. "A Randomized Trial of Two Different Doses of a SHR-5 Rhodiola Rosea Extract Versus Placebo and Control of Capacity for Mental Work." Phytomedicine. 2003 Mar; 10(2-3): 95-105.

Spasov A.A., et al. "A Double-blind, Placebo-controlled Pilot Study of the Stimulating and Adaptogenic Effect of Rhodiola Rosea SHR-5 Extract on the Fatigue of Students Caused by Stress During an Examination Period with a Repeated Low-dose Regimen." Phytomedicine. 2000 Apr; 7(2): 85-9.

Wilson J.L. Adrenal Fatigue: The 21st Century Stress Syndrome. Petaluma, CA: Smart Publications, 2001.

Halpin LS, et al. "Guided Imagery in Cardiac Surgery." Outcomes Manag. 2002 Jul-Sep; 6(3): 132-7.

Kline WH, et al. "Enhancing Pain Management in the PICU by Teaching Guided Mental Imagery: A Quality-Improvement Project." J Pediatr Psychol. 2009 Apr 22. [Epub ahead of print]

Weigensberg MJ, et al. "Acute Effects of Stress-Reduction Interactive Guided Imagery(SM) on Salivary Cortisol in Overweight Latino Adolescents." J Altern Complement Med. 2009 Mar; 15(3): 297-303.

Kemps E, and Tiggemann M. "Competing Visual and Olfactory Imagery Tasks Suppress Craving for Coffee." Exp Clin Psychopharmacol. 2009 Feb; 17(1): 43-50.

Eremin O, et al. "Immuno-modulatory Effects of Relaxation Training and Guided Imagery in Women with Locally Advanced Breast Cancer Undergoing Multimodality Therapy: A randomized Controlled Trial." Breast. 2009 Feb; 18(1): 17-25.

Liu KP, et al. "A Randomized Controlled Trial of Mental Imagery Augment Generalization of Learning in Acute Poststroke Patients." Stroke. 2009 Jun; 40(6): 2222-5.

Hayashi T, and Murakami K. "The Effects of Laughter on Post-prandial Glucose Levels and Gene Expression in Type 2 Diabetic Patients." Life Sci. 2009 Jul 31; 85(5-6): 185-7.

Miller M and Fry WF. "The Effect of Mirthful Laughter on the Human Cardiovascular System." Med Hypotheses. 2009 May 26. [Epub ahead of print]

Jancin B. "Pleasurable Lifestyle Changes Can Cut Cardiac Risk." Family Practice News. 1998 December 15:14-15.

Also by Lorna R. Vanderhaeghe

A Smart Woman's Guide to Hormones

A Smart Woman's Guide to Weight Loss

An A-Z Woman's Guide to Vibrant Health

A Smart Woman's Guide to Heart Health

Healthy Fats for Life:
Preventing and Treating Common Health
Problems with Essential Fatty Acids
with Karlene Karst, BSc, RD

Healthy Immunity:
Scientifically Proven Natural Treatments for
Conditions from A-Z

The Immune System Cure:
Nature's Way to Super-Powered Health
with Patrick JD Bouic, PhD

For more information about Lorna Vanderhaeghe, visit

www.hormonehelp.com

CALA-Q Plus™

Calamari DHA and EPA plus Q10 and Carnitine

What to expect from this product:

- ♥ Omega-3
- ♥ Supports a healthy heart
- ♥ Promotes normal blood pressure
- ♥ Lowers "bad" LDL cholesterol and raises "good" HDL cholesterol
- ♥ Normalizes C-reactive protein
- ♥ Vital for healthy eyes
- ♥ Contains calamari oil rich in DHA
- ♥ No fishy aftertaste or unpleasant "repeating"

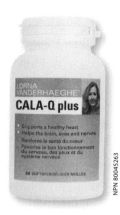

Potent Antioxidants: Calamari Marine Oils
Fish oils are well known for their heart-healthy effects. Containing the fatty acids EPA and DHA, fish oils, are vital to eye, brain and colon health. Calamari oil, an alternative to fish oil, comes from South American calamari (squid) that are sustainably harvested and an eco-friendly source of omega-3 fatty acids with more DHA than fish oil. DHA makes up 40 percent of the essential fats in your brain. Calamari oil is more stable than traditional fish oils, making it less prone to rancidity. Also, calamari oil does not cause the fish aftertaste or unpleasant "repeating" that is common with fish oil supplements. DHA is superior for lowering high blood pressure and it is more potent at supporting circulation. DHA is also the key to raising "good" HDL cholesterol. Also, DHA, not EPA,has been found to support your brain and is the best fatty acid for eye health. If you care about the environment calamari oil is your best choice as it comes from deep-water, spawns quickly, multiplies fast and does not have the same issues with heavy metals that fish do.

L-Carnitine Fumarate
Carnitine fumarate helps coenzyme Q10 do its job. Carnitine is a super antioxidant needed by your heart, brain cells and arteries. CALA-Q Plus contains the most absorbable form of carnitine as fumarate.

Coenzyme Q10
Coenzyme Q10 is found in almost every cell in the body. It is called the "Spark of Life" providing a powerful energy boost. People on statin medications should supplement with CoQ10 as this common group of cholesterol drugs depletes the body's CoQ10. CALA-Q Plus provides triple support for lowering blood pressure with the Calamari oil, CoQ10 and the additional B vitamins. Coenzyme Q10 has also been used to treat gum disease, which is linked to poor heart health. CALA-Q Plus contains a highly absorbable form of Q10.

Vitamin E
Vitamin E when combined with coenzyme Q10 keeps the "bad" LDL cholesterol from clogging up your arteries. Vitamin E is important in the prevention and

treatment of heart disease, cancer, Alzheimer's, menstrual pain, diabetes and rheumatoid arthritis.

Vitamin B6 (Pyridoxal-5-Phosphate)

CALA-Q Plus contains pyridoxal-5-phosphate the safest and most absorbable form of vitamin B6. Vitamin B6 is required for over 60 actions in the body including a healthy brain. Vitamin B6 helps the body make hormones such as serotonin and melatonin that influence mood and sleeping patterns. Symptoms of low vitamin B6 include muscle weakness, nervousness, irritability, depression, difficulty concentrating, and short-term memory loss.

Folic Acid

Folic acid works with vitamin B12 to control levels of the amino acid homocysteine. High levels of homocysteine are associated with heart disease. Folic acid also works with vitamin B12 to make red blood cells. Low levels of folic acid are common and can be caused by alcoholism, inflammatory bowel disease, celiac disease and certain medications. Folic acid along with vitamin B6 and vitamin B12 are essential for reducing the risk of heart disease.

Vitamin B12 (Methylcobalamin)

Seniors, vegetarians, vegans, and people with digestive issues and/or absorption problems are at particular risk of vitamin B12 deficiency. Vitamin B12 is used to treat pernicious anemia, heart disease, age-related macular degeneration and fatigue. Low vitamin B12 can cause fatigue, shortness of breath, nervousness, tingling in the extremities and numbness. CALA-Q Plus contains methylcobalamin, the most absorbable form of vitamin B12.

FORMULA:

EACH 2 SOFTGELS CONTAIN:

Calamari oil	1000 mg
DHA (Docosahexaenoic acid)	720 mg
EPA (Eicosapentaenoic acid)	280 mg
L-Carnitine (Fumarate)	200 mg
Coenzyme Q10 (Ubiquinone)	50 mg
Vitamin B6 (Pyridoxal-5-phosphate)	30 mg
Vitamin E (D-alpha tocopheryl acetate)	50 IU
Vitamin B12 (Methylcobalamin)	750 mcg
Folate (Folic acid)	400 mcg

Encapsulated in gelatin, glycerine, roasted carob powder, sunflower lecithin, beeswax and purified water.

This product does not contain artificial preservatives, colour or sweeteners; no corn, dairy, gluten, soy, wheat or yeast. **GLUTEN-FREE.**

SUGGESTED USAGE:

• Take 2 softgels once per day with food or as directed by a health care professional.